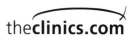

PEDIATRIC CLINICS
OF NORTH AMERICA

Children's Health and the Environment: Part I

GUEST EDITORS
Jerome A. Paulson, MD, FAAP
Benjamin A. Gitterman, MD, FAAP

February 2007 • Volume 54 • Number 1

SAUNDERS

An Imprint of Elsevier, Inc.
PHILADELPHIA   LONDON   TORONTO   MONTREAL   SYDNEY   TOKYO

W.B. SAUNDERS COMPANY
A Division of Elsevier Inc.

1600 John F. Kennedy Boulevard • Suite 1800 • Philadelphia, Pennsylvania 19103

http://www.theclinics.com

THE PEDIATRIC CLINICS OF NORTH AMERICA   Volume 54, Number 1
February 2007   ISSN 0031-3955
Editor: Carla Holloway   ISBN-13: 978-1-4160-4352-2
                                            ISBN-10: 1-4160-4352-7

The ideas and opinions expressed in *The Pediatric Clinics of North America* do not necessarily reflect those of the Publisher. The Publisher does not assume any responsibility for any injury and/or damage to persons or property arising out of or related to any use of the material contained in this periodical. The reader is advised to check the appropriate medical literature and the product information currently provided by the manufacturer of each drug to be administered to verify the dosage, the method and duration of adminis-tration, or contraindications. It is the responsibility of the treating physician or other health care profes-sional, relying on independent experience and knowledge of the patient, to determine drug dosages and the best treatment for the patient. Mention of any product in this issue should not be construed as endorse-ment by the contributors, editors, or the Publisher of the product or manufacturers' claims.

The Pediatric Clinics of North America (ISSN 0031-3955) is published bi-monthly by Elsevier Inc. 360 Park Avenue South, New York, NY 10010-1710. Months of publication are February, April, June, August, Octo-ber, and December. Business and Editorial Offices: 1600 John F. Kennedy Blvd., Suite 1800, Philadelphia, PA 19103-2899. Customer Service Office: 6277 Sea Harbor Drive, Orlando, FL 32887-4800. Periodicals post-age paid at New York, NY and additional mailing offices. Subscription prices are $138.00 per year (US in-dividuals), $281.00 per year (US institutions), $187.00 per year (Canadian individuals), $367.00 per year (Canadian institutions), $209.00 per year (international individuals), $367.00 per year (international institu-tions), $72.00 per year (US students), $110.00 per year (Canadian students), and $110.00 per year (foreign students). To receive students/resident rare, orders must be accompanied by name of affiliated institution, date of term, and the signature of program/residency coordinator on institution letterhead. Orders will be billed at individual rate until proof of status is received. Foreign air speed delivery is included in all Clinics subscription prices. All prices are subject to change without notice. POSTMASTER: Send address changes to *The Pediatric Clinics of North America*, Elsevier Periodicals Customer Service, 6277 Sea Harbor Drive, Orlando, FL 32887-4800. **Customer Service: 1-800-654-2452 (US). From outside of the US, call 1-407-345-4000**. E-mail: hhspcs@harcourt.com.

The Pediatric Clinics of North America is also published in Spanish by McGraw-Hill Inter-americana Editores S.A., Mexico City, Mexico; in Portuguese by Riechmann and Affonso Editores, Rua Comandante Coelho 1085, CEP 21250, Rio de Janeiro, Brazil; and in Greek by Althayia SA, Athens, Greece.

The Pediatric Clinics of North America is covered in *Index Medicus, Excerpta Medica, Current Contents, Current Contents/Clinical Medicine, Science Citation Index, ASCA, ISI/BIOMED*, and *BIOSIS*.

Printed in the United States of America.

GUEST EDITORS

JEROME A. PAULSON, MD, FAAP, Associate Professor of Pediatrics and Public Health, Co-Director, Mid-Atlantic Center for Children's Health and the Environment, George Washington University, Washington, District of Columbia

BENJAMIN A. GITTERMAN, MD, FAAP, Associate Professor of Pediatrics and Public Health, Co-Director, Mid-Atlantic Center for Children's Health and the Environment, George Washington University, Washington, District of Columbia

CONTRIBUTORS

STACEY J. ARNESEN, MS, Advisor for Special Projects, Specialized Information Services, National Library of Medicine, Bethesda, Maryland

JOHN M. BELMONT, PhD, Professor Emeritus, Department of Pediatrics, University of Kansas School of Medicine, Kansas City, Kansas

PATRICK BREYSSE, PhD, Professor, Department of Environmental Health Sciences, Johns Hopkins Bloomberg School of Public Health, Baltimore, Maryland

ALICE C. BROCK-UTNE, MD, Clinical Instructor, University of California at San Francisco, San Francisco, California

IRENA BUKA, MB, ChB, FRCPC, Paediatric Environmental Health Specialty Unit, Misericordia Hospital, Edmonton; and Department of Paediatrics, University of Alberta, Alberta, Canada

DEBRA C. CHERRY, MD, MS, Assistant Professor, Occupational Health Sciences, University of Texas Health Center at Tyler; Medical Director, Southwest Center for Pediatric Environmental Health; and Director, Texas Cancer Registry/East Texas Regional Office, Tyler, Texas

GREGORY B. DIETTE, MD, MHS, Associate Professor, Division of Pulmonary and Critical Care Medicine, Department of Medicine, Johns Hopkins University School of Medicine, Baltimore, Maryland

PEYTON EGGLESTON, MD, Professor, Division of Allergy and Immunology, Department of Pediatrics, Johns Hopkins University School of Medicine, Baltimore, Maryland

JOEL FORMAN, MD, Associate Professor, Department of Pediatrics, Department of Community and Preventive Medicine, Mount Sinai School of Medicine, New York, New York

MAIDA P. GALVEZ, MD, MPH, Assistant Professor, Department of Community and Preventive Medicine, Department of Pediatrics, Mount Sinai School of Medicine, New York, New York

KAREN GILMORE, MPH, Program Director, Southwest Center for Agricultural Health, Injury Prevention, and Education, University of Texas Health Center at Tyler; and Occupational Health Sciences, University of Texas Health Center at Tyler, Tyler, Texas

NATHAN GRABER, MD, MPH, Instructor, Department of Community and Preventive Medicine, Department of Pediatrics, Mount Sinai School of Medicine, New York, New York

NADIA N. HANSEL, MD, MPH, Instructor, Division of Pulmonary and Critical Care Medicine, Department of Medicine, Johns Hopkins University School of Medicine, Baltimore, Maryland

HOWARD HU, MD, MPH, ScD, Professor and Chair, Department of Environmental Health Sciences, University of Michigan School of Public Health, Ann Arbor, Michigan; Adjunct Professor of Occupational and Environmental Medicine, Department of Environmental Health, Harvard School of Public Health; and Associate Professor of Medicine, Channing Laboratory, Brigham and Women's Hospital, Harvard Medical School, Boston, Massachusetts

BARBARA HUGGINS, MD, Medical Consultant, Southwest Center for Pediatric Environmental Health; (formerly) Professor and Chair, Department of Pediatrics, University of Texas Health Center at Tyler, Tyler, Texas

JAVED HUSSAIN, MD, Fellow, Pediatric Environmental Health, Children's Hospital Boston; and Instructor, Harvard Medical School, Boston, Massachusetts

CATHERINE J. KARR, MD, PhD, MS, Assistant Professor (acting), Department of Pediatrics; Adjunct Assistant Professor, Department of Environmental & Occupational Health Sciences; and Director, Pediatric Environmental Health Specialty Unit, University of Washington, Seattle, Washington

KATHERINE H. KIRKLAND, MPH, Executive Director, Association of Occupational and Environmental Clinics, Washington, District of Columbia

SAMUEL KORANTENG, MB, ChB, Paediatric Environmental Health Specialty Unit, Misericordia Hospital, Edmonton, Alberta, Canada

JENNIFER A. LOWRY, MD, Assistant Professor, Department of Pediatrics, University of Kansas School of Medicine; Mid-America Pediatric Environmental Health Specialty Unit, Center for Occupational and Environmental Health, University of Kansas Medical Center; and Mid-America Poison Control Center, University of Kansas Medical Center, Kansas City, Kansas

ELIZABETH MATSUI, MD, MHS, Assistant Professor, Division of Allergy and Immunology, Department of Pediatrics, Johns Hopkins University School of Medicine, Baltimore, Maryland

MARK D. MILLER, MD, MPH, Director, UCSF Pediatric Environmental Health Specialty Unit; California Poison Control System; and Assistant Clinical Professor, Department of Pediatrics, University of California at San Francisco, San Francisco, California

KAREN B. MULLOY, DO, MSCH, Assistant Professor, Program in Occupational and Environmental Health, Department of Internal Medicine, University of New Mexico, Albuquerque, New Mexico; and President, Board of Directors, Association of Occupational and Environmental Clinics, Washington, District of Columbia

JEROME A. PAULSON, MD, FAAP, Associate Professor of Pediatrics and Public Health, Co-Director, Mid-Atlantic Center for Children's Health and the Environment, George Washington University, Washington, District of Columbia

RICHARD PETERS, DrPH, MBA, MSc, Center for Risk Communication, New York, New York

MEGAN SANDEL, MD, MPH, Staff Pediatrician, Pediatric Environmental Health Center, Children's Hospital Boston; and Assistant Professor, Boston University Medical Center, Boston, Massachusetts

MICHAEL W. SHANNON, MD, MPH, Professor, Harvard Medical School; Co-Director, Pediatric Environmental Health Subspecialty Unit, Children's Hospital Boston; Cambridge Hospital; and Division of Emergency Medicine, Children's Hospital Boston, Boston, Massachusetts

HEMANT P. SHARMA, MD, Fellow, Division of Allergy and Immunology, Department of Pediatrics, Johns Hopkins University School of Medicine, Baltimore, Maryland

JAMES SHINE, PhD, Associate Professor of Aquatic Chemistry, Department of Environmental Health, Harvard School of Public Health, Boston, Massachusetts

GINA M. SOLOMON, MD, MPH, Associate Clinical Professor, Division of Occupational and Environmental Medicine; University of California at San Francisco; Associate Director, Pediatric Environmental Health Specialty Unit, University of California at San Francisco; and Senior Scientist, Natural Resources Defense Council, San Francisco, California

JOSEF G. THUNDIYIL, MD, MPH, Assistant Clinical Professor, Department of Emergency Medicine, Orlando Regional Medical Center, Orlando, Florida; (formerly) Fellow, California Poison Control System; and Resident, Division of Occupational and Environmental Medicine, University of California at San Francisco, San Francisco, California

ALVARO R. OSORNIO VARGAS, MD, PhD, División de Investigación Básica, Instituto Nacional de Cancerología, Mexico City, Mexico

KATHRYN VEAL, MD, MPH, Clinical Assistant Professor, Department of Pediatrics, University of Kansas School of Medicine; and Mid-America Pediatric Environmental Health Specialty Unit, Center for Occupational and Environmental Health, University of Kansas Medical Center, Kansas City, Kansas

PAULA WILBORNE-DAVIS, MPH, CHES, Program Manager, PEHSU Program, Association of Occupational and Environmental Clinics, Washington, District of Columbia

ALAN D. WOOLF, MD, MPH, Associate Professor, Harvard Medical School; Co-Director, Pediatric Environmental Health Subspecialty Unit, Children's Hospital Boston; and Cambridge Hospital, Cambridge, Massachusetts

ROBERT O. WRIGHT, MD, MPH, Department of Environmental Health Sciences, University of Michigan School of Public Health, Ann Arbor, Michigan; Associate Professor, Center for Children's Environmental Health and Disease Prevention, Department of Environmental Health, Harvard School of Public Health; and Assistant Professor of Medicine, Channing Laboratory, Brigham and Women's Hospital, Harvard Medical School, Boston, Massachusetts

CONTRIBUTORS

CONTENTS

The unique biologic characteristics and behaviors of children make
them vulnerable to environmental toxicants. Physicians and other
health professionals are challenged in addressing pediatric environmental health care needs in part because of deficient knowledge and
skills in pediatric environmental health. This deficiency seems to stem
from inadequate exposure to the field of pediatric environmental
health during clinical training. The foundational goal of the PEHSU
program is to address the gap in pediatric environmental health
knowledge by enhancing the fundamental knowledge and skills of
pediatricians, primary care physicians, and other health professionals.

Currently, the only national databases that are available to aid in a
search to assess the effect of environmental exposures on children's
health are those provided by the Pediatric Environmental Health
Specialty Units and poison control centers. Both have limitations
and are largely deficient in accurate, helpful numbers. Both, however, offer insight into factors that are important to the public
and health care professionals and provide some outcome data to
measure morbidity and mortality. This article presents an analysis
of the information in these databases about children's exposure to
toxic environmental substances.

In situations with visible threats to children's health, pediatric health care providers must be prepared to communicate the health risks of environmental exposures. Several factors influence the effectiveness of such discussions: whether the individual providing the information is considered a reliable source, the familiarity of the physician and parent/guardian with these issues, and the limited research specifically assessing risk of exposure in childhood. This article describes the theory behind effective risk communication using examples from events following September 11, 2001. It shares lessons learned and provides a template for risk communication that can guide pediatric providers.

Children's health can be affected adversely by the environment in which they live. It is well recognized that some environmental chemicals are harmful to the brain, but the role these chemicals play in the development of specific disabilities such as attention deficit hyperactivity disorder and autism is not certain. Parents of children who have developmental disabilities often ask the primary care physician whether certain environmental toxicants might be the cause of the illness. A detailed environmental history and physical examination may help clarify whether there is a plausible relationship between an environmental toxicant and a child's disability.

Children encounter pesticide products and their residues where they live and play and in the food supply. Pesticide exposure affects pediatric health both acutely and chronically; effects range from mild and subtle to severe. Pediatricians play an important role in identifying and reducing significant pesticide exposure in their patients by taking an exposure history to clarify the extent and types of exposures that may have occurred during acute care and preventive care visits. Developing knowledge about the toxicity of various chemicals, identifying reliable resources for pesticide information, and providing a common-sense approach toward recommending the safest practical alternatives is necessary.

information and discusses how to evaluate such information. It also provides an extensive list of environmental-health-related websites hosted by governmental and nongovernmental agencies, and other organizations.

In the United States, many of the millions of tons of hazardous wastes that have been produced since World War II have accumulated in sites throughout the nation. Citizen concern about the extent of this problem led Congress to establish the Superfund Program in 1980 to locate, investigate, and clean up the worst sites nationwide. Most such waste exists as a complex mixture of many substances. This article discusses the issue of toxic mixtures and children's health by focusing on the specific example of mining waste at the Tar Creek Superfund Site in Northeast Oklahoma.

Cancer in children is rare and accounts for about 1% of all malignancies. In the developed world, however, it is the commonest cause of disease-related deaths in childhood, carrying with it a great economic and emotional cost. Cancers are assumed to be multivariate, multifactorial diseases that occur when a complex and prolonged process involving genetic and environmental factors interact in a multistage sequence. This article explores the available evidence for this process, primarily from the environmental linkages perspective but including some evidence of the genetic factors.

PEDIATRIC CLINICS OF NORTH AMERICA FEBRUARY 2007

GOAL STATEMENT
The goal of *Pediatric Clinics of North America* is to keep practicing physicians and residents up to date with current clinical practice in pediatrics by providing timely articles reviewing the state-of-the-art in patient care.

ACCREDITATION
The *Pediatric Clinics of North America* is planned and implemented in accordance with the Essential Areas and Policies of the Accreditation Council for Continuing Medical Education (ACCME) through the joint sponsorship of the University Of Virginia School Of Medicine and Elsevier. The University Of Virginia School of Medicine is accredited by the ACCME to provide continuing medical education for physicians.

The University of Virginia School of Medicine designates this educational activity for a maximum of 15 *AMA PRA Category 1 Credits*™. Physicians should only claim credit commensurate with the extent of their participation in the activity.

The American Medical Association has determined that physicians not licensed in the US who participate in this CME activity are eligible for 15 *AMA PRA Category 1 Credits*.™

Credit can be earned by reading the text material, taking the CME examination online at http://www.theclinics.com/home/cme, and completing the evaluation. After taking the test, you will be required to review any and all incorrect answers. Following completion of the test and evaluation, your credit will be awarded and you may print your certificate.

FACULTY DISCLOSURE/CONFLICT OF INTEREST
The University of Virginia School of Medicine, as an ACCME accredited provider, endorses and strives to comply with the Accreditation Council for Continuing Medical Education (ACCME) Standards of Commercial Support, Commonwealth of Virginia statutes, University of Virginia policies and procedures, and associated federal and private regulations and guidelines on the need for disclosure and monitoring of proprietary and financial interests that may affect the scientific integrity and balance of content delivered in continuing medical education activities under our auspices.

The University of Virginia School of Medicine requires that all CME activities accredited through this institution be developed independently and be scientifically rigorous, balanced and objective in the presentation/discussion of its content, theories and practices.

All authors/editors participating in an accredited CME activity are expected to disclose to the readers relevant financial relationships with commercial entities occurring within the past 12 months (such as grants or research support, employee, consultant, stock holder, member of speakers bureau, etc.). The University of Virginia School of Medicine will employ appropriate mechanisms to resolve potential conflicts of interest to maintain the standards of fair and balanced education to the reader. Questions about specific strategies can be directed to the Office of Continuing Medical Education, University of Virginia School of Medicine, Charlottesville, Virginia.

The authors/editors listed below have identified no financial or professional relationships for themselves or their spouse/partner: Stacey J. Arneson, MLS; John M. Belmont, PhD; Patrick Breysse, PhD; Alice C. Brock-Utne, MD; Irena Buka, MBChB, FRCPC; Debra C. Cherry, MD; Gregory B. Diette, MD, MHS; Joel Forman, MD; M.H. Frumkin, MD, MPH; Maida Galvez, MD, MPH; Karen Gilmore, MPH; Benjamin A. Gitterman, MD (Guest Editor); Nathan M. Graber, MD; Nadia Hansel, MDm MPH; Carla Holloway (Acquisitions Editor); Howard Hu, MD, MPH, ScD; Barbara W. Huggins, MD; Javed H. Hussain, MD; Catherine Karr, MD, PhD; Katherine H. Kirkland, MPH; Samuel Koranteng, MB, ChB; Jennifer A. Lowry, MD; Elizabeth Matsui, MD, MHS; Mark D. Miller, MD, MPH; Megan Sandel, MD; Michael W. Shannon, MD, MPH; Hemant P. Sharma, MD; James Shine, PhD; Gina M. Solomon, MD, MPH; Josef G. Thundiyil, MD, MPH; Alvaro R. Osornio Vargas, MD, PhD; Kathryn Veal, MD, MPH; Paula Wilborne-Davis, MPH, CHES; Alan D. Woolf, MD, MPH; and, Robert O. Wright, MD, MPH.

The authors/editors listed below identified the following professional or financial affiliations for themselves or their spouse/partner:
Peyton A. Eggleston, MD is a consultant for Proctor and Gamble, S C Johnson, and Church and Dwight.
Karen Mulloy DO, MSCD is a principal investigator or co-investigator for NIOSH, HRSA, and AOEC/ATSDR.
Jerome A. Paulson, MD, FAAP (Guest Editor) owns stock in renal Ventures Ltd, Dialysis.
Richard G. Peters, DrPH, MBA, MSc is a consultant for the Center for Risk Communication.

Disclosure of Discussion of Non-FDA Approved Uses for Pharmaceutical and/or Medical Devices.
The University of Virginia School of Medicine, as an ACCME provider, requires that all authors identify and disclose any "off label" uses for pharmaceutical and medical device products. The University of Virginia School of Medicine recommends that each physician fully review all the available data on new products or procedures prior to clinical use.

TO ENROLL
To enroll in the Pediatric Clinics of North America Continuing Medical Education program, call customer service at 1-800-654-2452 or visit us online at www.theclinics.com/home/cme. The CME program is available to subscribers for an additional fee of $195.00.

FORTHCOMING ISSUES

RECENT ISSUES

ELSEVIER
SAUNDERS

Pediatr Clin N Am
54 (2007) xiii–xiv

PEDIATRIC CLINICS

OF NORTH AMERICA

Preface

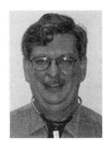
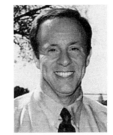

Jerome A. Paulson, MD, FAAP   Benjamin A. Gitterman, MD, FAAP
Guest Editors

Children's environmental health is one of the up-and-coming challenges of the twenty-first century. Palfrey and colleagues [1] have coined the term "millennial morbidities" to describe the most pressing new morbidities of our time—disorders of the bioenvironmental interface, socioeconomic influences on health, health disparities, technological influences on health, overweight and obesity, and mental health issues. In the last century the progress in the treatment of previously identified health care problems in many pediatric subspecialties, although hardly complete, has been spectacular. We now are in an era in which factors that affect the health of children increasingly are identified before the damage is evident, as evidenced by our increasing abilities to identify prenatal and genetically based conditions. Similarly, the impacts of environmental exposures are being understood, and, perhaps more importantly, are being recognized by larger segments of the health professional community and the public alike. Pediatricians now have a responsibility to improve their recognition and understanding of these exposures and to assess and communicate to others the potential risks and threats that environmental exposures pose to children. Finally, this increased understanding underscores the increasing need for pediatricians to be able to act on behalf of children and to do so through increased familiarity with and access to resources that can be of practical benefit to doctors and patients alike.

The *Pediatric Clinics of North America* first published an issue on children's environmental health in 2001. New and increasingly sophisticated information in this field is already available. Expanded resources now exist

0031-3955/07/$ - see front matter © 2007 Elsevier Inc. All rights reserved.
doi:10.1016/j.pcl.2007.01.001   *pediatric.theclinics.com*

to support child health professionals. The previous publication thoughtfully addressed many of the more obvious and traditional subjects in this field, for the first time in one volume. In this and the next issue of *Pediatric Clinics of North America*, we offer a collection of articles that address a wider range of environmental health issues that impact children in a number of settings as well as a discussion of issues that the public may be bring to us as health professionals.

At the time of the original publication, the Pediatric Environmental Health Specialty Units were just getting organized. Now a network of 12 units serves all regions of the United States as well as much of North America. Individuals from these units form the core of the group of authors for these issues of *Pediatric Clinics*. The expertise in each of the units individually and in all of the units cumulatively is exceedingly broad and serves as an important resource for education and clinical consultation.

The other articles in this issue of *Pediatric Clinics* are drawn from several of the Centers for Children's Environmental Health and Disease Prevention Research located throughout the country. These centers are the research engine in the nascent but rapidly expanding field of children's health and the environment.

These new collections of articles should be highly relevant to the knowledge and work of medical, nursing, and public health professionals involved in all realms and specialties of pediatric health.

Jerome A. Paulson, MD, FAAP
Associate Professor of Pediatrics and Public Health
Co-Director, Mid-Atlantic Center for Children's Health and the Environment
George Washington University
2100 M Street NW, Suite 203
Washington, DC 20052, USA

E-mail address: jpaulson@cnmc.org

Benjamin A. Gitterman, MD, FAAP
Associate Professor of Pediatrics and Public Health
Co-Director, Mid-Atlantic Center for Children's Health and the Environment
George Washington University
2100 M Street NW, Suite 203
Washington, DC 20052, USA

E-mail address: bgitterm@cnmc.org

Reference

[1] Palfrey JS, Tonniges TF, Green M, et al. Introduction: addressing the millennial morbidity—the context of community pediatrics. Pediatrics 2005;115(4 Suppl):1121–3.

ELSEVIER
SAUNDERS

Pediatr Clin N Am
54 (2007) xv

PEDIATRIC CLINICS
OF NORTH AMERICA

Dedication

This issue is dedicated to Gwen Paulson and to Anna, Robert and Sara Gitterman. It also is dedicated to the women and men who work tirelessly to improve the environment for children—those in the Office of Children's Health Protection and the rest of the US Environmental Protection Agency (EPA), as well as the Agency for Toxic Substances and Disease Registry (ATSDR) along with the rest of the Centers for Disease Control and Prevention (CDC). They are striving to create a healthier, safer future for the children of today and for generations to come.

Jerome A. Paulson, MD, FAAP
Benjamin A. Gitterman, MD, FAAP

0031-3955/07/$ - see front matter © 2007 Elsevier Inc. All rights reserved.
doi:10.1016/j.pcl.2007.01.002
pediatric.theclinics.com

ELSEVIER
SAUNDERS

Pediatr Clin N Am
54 (2007) 1–13

PEDIATRIC CLINICS

OF NORTH AMERICA

A Model for Physician Education and Consultation in Pediatric Environmental Health—The Pediatric Environmental Health Specialty Units (PEHSU) Program

Paula Wilborne-Davis, MPH, CHES,
Katherine H. Kirkland, MPH*,
Karen B. Mulloy, DO, MSCH[1]

*Association of Occupational and Environmental Clinics, 1010 Vermont Avenue,
NW, Suite 513, Washington, DC 20005, USA*

Children have unique vulnerabilities to environmental exposures because of their different metabolism, body structure, daily behavior, and lifestyle. They come in contact, often unknowingly, with environmental hazards during their daily activities at school, at work, and at play. For example, for a child who has asthma, going to chemistry class may trigger asthmatic symptoms that require the child to visit the school nurse frequently. When attending other classrooms in the school, however, the child has no symptoms. The parents become concerned and take the child to the family pediatrician. The pediatrician is puzzled as to why these symptoms only occur at chemistry class. As part of the pediatric environmental history, the pediatrician asks the child what type of chemistry experiments are being conducted in the class and the types of chemicals being used. It is discovered that one of the chemicals is a known asthmagen. The pediatrician notifies the school administrator to recommend that this particular chemical be

The PEHSU program is funded by the Agency for Toxic Substances and Disease Registry, Cooperative Agreement U50/ATU374312 and the U.S. Environmental Protection Agency.

* Corresponding author.

[1] Present address: University of New Mexico School of Medicine, MSC10 5550, 1 University of New Mexico, Albuquerque, NM 87131-0001, USA.

E-mail address: kkirkland@aoec.org (K.H. Kirkland).

doi:10.1016/j.pcl.2006.11.001

removed from use by the patient and other students. This situation demonstrates the importance of the health care provider's knowledge and ability to incorporate a pediatric environmental history when symptoms and illnesses may be linked to an environmental cause [1].

In a sample survey of practicing pediatricians in Georgia, it was determined that pediatricians have a great interest in pediatric environmental health but lack the confidence in their ability to take a pediatric environmental history. The lack of proficiency in this skill maybe related to the fact that only one of five of the physicians in the survey had any training in environmental history taking [2].

The foundation and mission of the Pediatric Environmental Health Specialty Units (PEHSU) program is to provide education and consultation for health care providers, public health professionals, and others about the topic of children's environmental health. PEHSU sites also are involved in the education of the next generation of children's environmental health specialists through educational programs directed at medical students, pediatric residents, student nurses, and pediatric environmental health fellows.

The Pediatric Environmental Health Specialty Units program background/history

Two major environmental exposure incidents in 1996 served as the catalysts in the creation of the PEHSU program. Methyl parathion (an organophosphate insecticide) was used illegally inside homes in areas of Illinois, Mississippi, and Ohio to kill cockroaches and other insects. Entire families were exposed, including many children. Methyl parathion is designed only for outside use and is extremely toxic.

In another incident, a former warehouse in New Jersey, where fluorescent lights were previously manufactured, was converted into apartments. The manufacturing process involved mercury that had been poorly controlled in the building. More than a dozen families and their children were exposed to mercury from the contamination left in the building.

In both incidents, the majority of physicians providing care to the families had difficulty in recognizing the relationship of the environmental exposures in the affected children. With these events in mind, in 1996 the Agency for Toxic Substances and Disease Registry (ATSDR) launched the Child Health Initiative. The purpose of the initiative was to address the environmental health of children and the need for clinically based programs to evaluate potential adverse health effects of environmental exposures in children [3].

In 1998, as part of this ongoing effort, the ATSDR established the PEHSU program through a cooperative agreement with the Association of Occupational and Environmental Clinics (AOEC), a nonprofit organization committed to improving the practice of occupational and environmental health through information sharing and collaborative research. The program was developed to serve as a national resource for health care providers, state, federal, and local government officials, and the public.

The PEHSU program is comprised of a nationwide network of 11 sites in the United States that provide services to a defined geographic area including three or more states (Fig. 1). Additionally the network includes two international sites, one in Canada and one in Mexico. Table 1 lists the sites and their respective contact information. The framework for each PEHSU site is comprised of a formal collaboration between the Occupational and Environmental Medicine clinic (which is an AOEC clinic member) and the academic or medical center–based pediatric department within the same institution. The basic staffing structure includes board-certified pediatricians and board-certified occupational and environmental medicine physicians providing oversight of the programmatic and financial aspects. A project coordinator manages the daily operational issues. The PEHSU staffing structure is designed to incorporate multidisciplinary health professionals. Through formal agreements with other departments within the medical institution, access to toxicologists, allergists, pediatric neurologists, and other health care providers exist. Referrals to these departments and other health care professionals with specialties that are relevant to pediatric environmental health

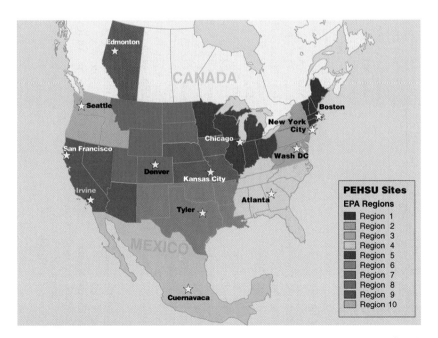

Fig. 1. Pediatric Environmental Health Specialty Units sites. (*From* U.S. Department of Health and Human Services. Agency for Toxic Substances and Disease Registry. Pediatric Environmental Health Specialty Units (PEHSU). Available at: http://www.atsdr.cdc.gov/HEC/natorg/pehsu.html).

Table 1
Pediatric Environmental Health Specialty Units regional locations and contact information*

Name	Location and Region Covered	Telephone Number and Website
New England Pediatric Environmental Health Specialty Unit	Boston, MA; EPA region I: CT, MA, ME, NH, RI, VT	1-888-244-5314; 617-355-8177 (local) www.childrenshospital.org/pehc
Mount Sinai Pediatric Environmental Health Specialty Unit	New York, NY; EPA region II: NJ, NY, PR, VI	1-866-265-6201 www.mssm.edu/cpm/peds_environ.shtml
The Mid-Atlantic Center for Children's Health & the Environment	Washington, DC; EPA region III: District of Columbia, DE, MD, PA, VA, WV	1-866-622-2431; 202-994-1166 (local) www.health-e-kids.org
The Southeast Pediatric Environmental Health Specialty Unit	Atlanta, GA; EPA region IV: AL, GA, FL, KY, MS, NC, SC, TN	1-877-337-3478; 404-727-9428 (local) www.sph.emory.edu/PEHSU
Great Lakes Center for Children's Environmental Health	Chicago, IL; EPA region V: IL, IN, MI, MN, OH, WI	1-800-672-3113; 312-864-5520 (local) www.uic.edu/sph/glakes/kids
Southwest Center for Pediatric Environmental Health	Tyler, TX; EPA region VI: AR, LA, NM, OK, TX	1-888-901-5665 www.swcpeh.org
The MidAmerica Pediatric Environmental Health Specialty Unit	Kansas City, KS; EPA region VII: IA, KS, MO, NE	1-800-421-9916; 913-588-6638 (local) www2.kumc.edu/mapehsu
Rocky Mountain Region–Pediatric Environmental Health Specialty Unit	Denver, CO; EPA region VIII: CO, SD, MT, ND, UT, WY	1-877-800-5554, www.rmrpehsu.org
The University of California Pediatric Environmental Health Specialty Unit	Irvine & San Francisco, CA; EPA region IX: AZ, CA, HI, NV	1-866-827-3478, University of California–Irvine, 949-824-1857 (local) www.coeh.uci.edu/pehsu University of California–San Francisco, 415-206-4083 (local), www.ucsf.edu/ucpehsu/
Northwest Pediatric Environmental Health Specialty Unit	Seattle, WA; EPA region X: AK, ID, OR, WA	1-877-543-2436, 206-744-9380 (local), http://depts.washington.edu/pehsu
Pediatric Environmental Health Clinic Misericordia Child Health Center	Edmonton, AB (Canada)	780-735-2731, email: mchhc.enviro@cha.ab.ca
Unidad Pediatrica Ambiental – Mexico Pediatric Environmental Helath Specialty Unit	Cuernavaca, Morelos (Mexico)	01-800-001-7777 (toll free Mexico only): 52-777-102-1259 (outside Mexico), www.upa-pehsu.org

* Information subject to change without notice. For latest information or further information contact AOEC at 1-888-347-2632 or aoec@aoec.org.

are also available. Although the operational structure is the same at each PEHSU site, each site has unique characteristics and expertise based on the environmental health needs and concerns of its defined geographic region. This expertise makes the PEHSU program a unique and valued resource in pediatric environmental health.

Goals and services

The ultimate goal of the PEHSU program is to increase the knowledge of pediatricians and other health care providers concerning pediatric environmental health. The three focal areas of the PEHSU program are education, consultation, and referral for children who may have been exposed to environmental hazards. Education is provided to various audiences, including practicing physicians attending major professional conferences, medical and nursing students during didactic, required class lectures, and formal continuing education opportunities.

Additionally, PEHSU staff provides community-based educational events to the general public. These events are primarily health fairs, community meetings, and school-related activities. The awareness of the importance of children's environmental health by the general public, especially parents, has increased significantly, and environmental health is listed as a top health concern by parents [4]. It is inferred that this phenomenon may be as a result of increased discussion of environmental health concerns of children by the media along with greater access to the Internet by the general public to obtain information related to pediatric environmental health.

An important service of the PEHSU sites is direct access to environmental health specialists. All of the PEHSU sites are required to have a toll-free telephone number dedicated to pediatric environmental health inquiries. This mechanism allows immediate access to PEHSU services for callers within the designated multistate geographic region. At 4 of the 11 sites, there is 24-hour, 7-day access with PEHSU calls screened by the local poison control center staff, who forward the information to the PEHSU. The PEHSU staff then contacts the caller to provide more in-depth response to the caller's concern. At most of the PEHSU sites, web sites further broaden access to PEHSU services. Inquiries can be sent by electronic mail, and responses by PEHSU staff can address specific problems while ensuring patient confidentiality.

The availability of clinical information and expert consultation between the PEHSU staff and health care providers is the program's core component for the clinician seeking advice. PEHSU staff is available to share its expertise in pediatric environmental health with practicing clinicians, health professionals in government agencies, and the community. With convenient access, clinicians are able to contact their regional PEHSU site during clinic practice hours. According to a 2005 marketing survey of a sample of the PEHSU stakeholders, the availability of free clinical consultations was ranked number one as a "unique and valuable" service provided by the PEHSU program. This service also was one of the most frequently used services [5].

Parents who contact a regional PEHSU site are encouraged to have the child's pediatrician/physician contact the PEHSU site directly for medical consultation with a pediatric environmental health specialist. By doing this, parents improve the health care provided their own child and improve the clinician's ability to provide better care to patients who have similar environmental health problems. Thus the clinician's pediatric environmental health knowledge and skills are enhanced based on specific clinical and diagnostic needs of their medical practice.

Educational focus

With the complex health care delivery system in the United States, children receive medical services from a variety of health care professionals in addition to the pediatrician. The primary goal of the PEHSU program is to enhance the knowledge of pediatricians and also of general physicians and other health care providers. To promote and sustain the profession of pediatric environmental medicine, it is critical to incorporate pediatric environmental health topics into medical training programs. Currently, educational opportunities in pediatric environmental medicine for residents in pediatric training programs and for medical and nursing students are minimal [6].

To meet this educational gap, the PEHSU staff at all sites emphasizes the provision of knowledge through consultation with practicing clinicians and clinical trainees in community-based and academic settings. The venues for reaching the target audiences vary to meet the needs of the audience. To reach practicing clinicians, PEHSU staff provides presentations at conferences, professional society meetings, medical grand rounds at hospitals, and individual medical consultations. Clinical trainees are served primarily in the academic setting with lectures during didactic courses. Topics for the educational presentations are selected to meet the needs of the audience and are relevant to the pediatric population being served.

In 2004, a review and analysis was performed of educational and outreach activities conducted by PEHSU staff for the period from July 2002 to June 2003 (n = 278). The data indicated that 73% of the PEHSU educational activities were conducted for practicing clinicians and health professionals. Clinical trainees were the target audience for 27% of the educational activities conducted. A review of the topics presented during the educational activities indicated that most of the topics were the same for practicing clinicians and clinical trainees. Some of the topics included were lead poisoning, asthma, and general introductory topics in pediatric environmental health such as "How to Take a Pediatric Environmental Health History" [7]. Often the topics presented for the clinicians were requested by the sponsoring institution or agency.

Impact of the Pediatric Environmental Health Specialty Units program on clinicians' education

Based on data collected from the PEHSU program quarterly reports, more than 23,000 clinicians and other health professionals received education from PEHSU staff from October 2004 to September 2005, based on more than 800 educational activities conducted. The clinician category includes physicians, nurse practitioners, medical faculty, nurses, and physician assistants; the health professional category includes other clinical and non-clinical professionals (eg, industrial hygienists), local health officials, and federal government staff at health agencies. (Fig. 2). The venue for these activities included conferences and association meetings reaching a large number of professionals. Lectures and presentations at medical facilities and community meetings were conducted also. In addition, PEHSU staff provided individual and small-group consultations. In an effort to reach a larger and more diverse audience, PEHSU staff served as guest speakers on television and radio shows.

For many clinicians in training and those in practice, the didactic and clinical information received from the PEHSU program has been the primary source of pediatric environmental health knowledge. Offering educational activities to practicing physicians in the community is challenging. For example, physicians in private practice often do not have the time to leave their busy solo practices to attend continuing education seminars. For many of the children affected by environmental exposure, however, the community-based health provider is their first point of contact with medical care.

The American Water Works Association Research Foundation conducted a research project on the risk of drinking water contamination as

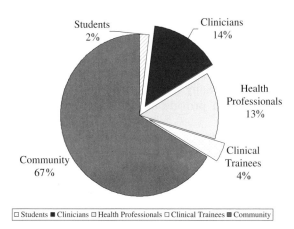

☐ Students ■ Clinicians ☐ Health Professionals ☐ Clinical Trainees ■ Community

Fig. 2. Outreach and education activities by target audience.

it related to physician communication with local health department and water utility staff. The research team conducted a survey of 30 clinicians along with a series of focus groups with seven physicians from across the United States who had primarily community-based family medicine practices. The community-based physicians provided suggestions on preferred mechanisms for receiving specific patient care medical information. The study found that community physicians want the information to be provided quickly and specific to their needs; it is best provided by telephone, fax, or electronic mail. The physicians preferred that information/education be provided by another physician who is knowledgeable about the subject to allow better communication and comprehension (ie, "both speaking the same language"). They also cited a need for appropriate patient education materials for distribution to patients. The group also discussed the inadequacies of their medical school training related to drinking water as a public and environmental health issue [8]. Many new findings in the environmental health field have been discovered in the last 20 years. The physicians in the focus group who attended medical school more than 20 years ago acknowledged that their skills and knowledge needed enhancement [8]. Similarly, in a study of community-based pediatricians, the American Academy of Pediatrics materials were the most widely recognized source for children environmental health information. Other sources included professional literature, government agencies, mass media, and colleagues' opinion [2]. Both groups preferred to receive clinical information from their peers.

To address the barriers related to communication with physicians, the PEHSU staff often uses existing community collaborative relationships to provide education to community-based physicians and other health professionals. Local health agencies and health departments consult with the PEHSU staff to assist in providing education to health professionals and the general public in the event of community-wide environmental exposures that affect children and their families. In this capacity, PEHSU staff is able to educate health care providers at health department–sponsored events including town meetings (held after office hours), weekend continuing education offerings, and specific ad hoc committee meetings in the community. PEHSU staff provides fundamental and clinical information specific to the environmental exposure of concern, meeting clinicians' immediate needs to provide care to potentially affected children. Events sponsored by the local medical association provide an additional mechanism for reaching community physicians.

The collective knowledge and expertise provided by the nationwide network of physicians, educators, and health professionals in the PEHSU program creates a unique arena for promoting and advancing the field of pediatric environmental health. Physicians and other health professionals use this network to discuss emerging issues and research in pediatric environmental health. At least three times a year, a "hot topics" conference call is conducted in which PEHSU staff and other health professionals discuss research and clinical approaches to emerging pediatric environmental health topics such as dioxins, mold health effects, autism, and other environmental exposure topics. Actual case studies based on clients receiving services at PEHSU sites are discussed also. The conference calls are facilitated by PEHSU staff or colleagues with shared expertise in pediatric environmental health.

Clinical trainee education and the Pediatric Environmental Health Specialty Units program

The education in pediatric environmental health provided by PEHSU staff is vital to enhancing the pediatric environmental knowledge of clinical trainees. For the period from October 2004 to September 30, 2005, PEHSU staff provided pediatric environmental health education to more than 3,000 clinical trainees as part of the 800 educational events conducted by PEHSU staff (see Fig. 2). The clinical trainees' category includes medical and nursing students, medical residents, and clinical fellows. To reach this audience, the educational events and lectures were conducted primarily in academic settings. In addition, the PEHSU staff provided individual mentoring and small-group sessions for trainees.

Because of the complexity of the health care delivery system in the United States, children receive medical services from a variety of health care professionals in addition to the pediatrician. To promote and sustain the profession of pediatric environmental medicine, it is critical to incorporate curriculum on pediatric environmental health into medical training programs. A curriculum that is built on competency-based learning objectives in environmental medicine such as those recommended by the Institute of Medicine's report, "Environmental Medicine: Integrating a Missing Element into Medical Education" [9]. Educational opportunities in pediatric environmental health for all medical trainees are minimal. In medical schools, environmental health education (as part of Occupational and Environmental Medicine) is generally limited to 4 hours over 4 years [6]. Typically the curriculum includes only a few lectures related to childhood lead poisoning and environmental triggers of asthma.

The foci of the clinical trainees' pediatric environmental health education should be to increase the awareness of the clinical impact related to environmental exposures in children, discuss vulnerable periods of child development and its relationship to the unique vulnerability of children, and discuss why the impact of environmental exposure is different for children than for adults. Accordingly, it is suggested that core knowledge should include an overview of stages of child development and its relationship to environmental exposures, how to take a pediatric environmental history, and the clinical impact of various environmental exposures.

The provision of this education/knowledge content is hindered also by the shortage of faculty in academically based pediatric departments that have pediatric environmental medicine knowledge. As in medical school, pediatric residency training programs generally limit pediatric environmental health education to a few topics unless a patient presents with an obvious environmental exposure. The lack of faculty with knowledge or expertise in pediatric environmental health can limit the educational and training opportunities for students [10].

To address this deficiency in environmental medicine faculty, all the PEHSU sites are located within academic medical institutions with PEHSU physicians as faculty members. This strategic location affords the PEHSU staff opportunities to provide lectures, mentoring and direct clinical/patient education to medical students, residents, and fellows as part of their didactic experiences.

The commitment of the PEHSU program to advancing the field of pediatric environmental medicine is exemplified by the involvement of staff in the various pediatric environmental health fellowships. In 2001 the Ambulatory Pediatric Association established the Pediatric Environmental Health Scholars program that provides specialized postresidency training in pediatric environmental medicine. The PEHSU sites currently have appointments for eight pediatric environmental health fellows. Financial sponsorship of the fellows is provided by a variety of sources (eg, the Ambulatory Pediatric Association, the National Institute of Environmental Health Sciences, and other agencies).

The impact of this experience and knowledge gained by the fellows is demonstrated in the integral involvement of the fellows in providing PEHSU services. A primary service of the PEHSU program is responding to telephone inquiries and consultation in which the fellows have a vital role. Additionally, the fellows provide direct patient care to children who have environmental illnesses, provide education and consultation to physicians and other health professionals, and are involved in pediatric environmental health research.

Duplication of the Pediatric Environmental Health Specialty Units model

There is a great deal of interest in the United States regarding the PEHSU model. Medical institutions in Connecticut, Iowa, and southern Ohio have communicated with the AOEC regarding the establishment of new PEHSU sites. In addition, the leadership at the Mount Sinai Pediatric Environmental Health Specialty Unit (in New York City) is working with state legislative personnel regarding establishment of satellite pediatric environmental health sites throughout the state of New York.

The PEHSU program network has expanded outside the United States with the Pediatric Environmental Health Clinic located in Alberta, Canada, and the Unidad Pediatrica Ambiental–Pediatric Environmental Health Specialty Unit located in Cuernavaca, Mexico. The involvement of the Canada PEHSU in the program is a formal collaboration with the United

States PEHSU network, but the Canadian site receives no funding from the United States. The Mexican Unidad Pediatrica Ambiental currently is funded by the US Environmental Protection Agency (EPA) through an AOEC agreement with the ATSDR. Both sites use the PEHSU model of staffing and operation while implementing the PEHSU program goals and services. The prevalent environmental health concerns in these two countries in most cases mirror those in the United States. Internationally, there has been interest expressed to the AOEC and the EPA Office of Children's Health Protection to establish PEHSU sites in several South American countries, including: Chile, Bolivia, Argentina, and Brazil. Additional sites in Mexico also have expressed interest in joining the existing network. The PEHSU, Great Lakes Center for Children's Environmental Health (located in Chicago) has begun working with clinicians in the Ukraine to establish a similar program. A program has been established in Spain based on the PEHSU model but is focused on the environmental impact of childhood cancer as the primary outcome of interest. In the establishment of these additional sites, care must be taken to ensure that the new PEHSU sites have the requisite levels of expertise in pediatrics, toxicology, and occupational medicine as part of their staffing or collaborative agreements. The synergy of these different specialties ensures the quality of the PEHSU network.

Future directions

The PEHSU program has a commitment to continue to focus on educational activities for physicians and clinical trainees by expanding and modifying existing approaches while adding more effective methods for reaching these target audiences. Future educational activities will be developed with consideration of the diverse needs of both of these audience segments.

In the the 2005 PEHSU marketing survey, PEHSU colleagues and stakeholders indicated a need for new or improved educational services to physicians and other health professionals. Regarding short-term education and training, it was suggested that web-based, self-paced instruction and webcast sessions be offered. In addition, recommendations were made regarding the use of the Internet to provide an online database of referral resources in pediatric environmental health. The development of a central PEHSU website with fact sheets and other educational resources related to prevalent and emerging pediatric environmental health issues would provide a single point of contact for health professionals. With an emphasis on clinical trainees, the results also indicated an interest in the PEHSU program continuing to offer pediatric environmental health fellowships [5].

The PEHSU program has embodied these suggestions in its goals for future programs. It has been determined that these approaches will allow a larger number of physicians and other health professionals to be reached and to access vital information at their convenience. Providing direct educational activities will continue to be a major feature of the PEHSU program.

Summary

The unique biologic characteristics and behaviors of children make them vulnerable to environmental toxicants. Physicians and other health professionals are challenged in addressing pediatric environmental health care needs, in part because of deficient knowledge and skills in pediatric environmental health. This deficiency seems to stem from inadequate exposure to the field of pediatric environmental health during their clinical training.

The foundational goal of the PEHSU program is to address the gap in pediatric environmental health knowledge by enhancing the fundamental knowledge and skills of pediatricians, primary care physicians, and other health professionals. The PEHSU program's network of pediatric environmental health specialists provides focused education and medical consultation to practicing clinicians and clinical trainees. Providing general education and clinical information about pertinent and emerging topics and issues in pediatric environmental health is the emphasis of the educational activities provided by the PEHSU staff.

The use of the Internet and other technology-based venues has become an essential tool in providing education and information to practicing clinicians and clinical trainees. The PEHSU program will incorporate this approach to reach a greater number of health professionals while providing convenient access.

The field of pediatric environmental health is increasingly recognized and accepted as a vital aspect of health care for children. The PEHSU program is committed to being a champion in this emerging field by providing training and education to current and future clinicians.

Acknowledgments

The authors thank Adam Spanier, MD, Iris G. Udasin, MD, and Tracey Delaney for their critical review of the manuscript.

References

[1] Etzel RA, Balk SJ. Handbook of pediatric environmental health. 2nd edition. Elk Grove Village (IL): American Academy of Pediatrics; 2003. p. 37.
[2] Kilpatrick N, Frumkin H, Trowbridge J, et al. The environmental history in pediatric practice: a study of pediatricians' attitudes, beliefs and practices. Environ Health Perspect 2002;110(8):823–7.
[3] Agency for Toxic Substances and Disease Registry (ATSDR). Healthy children—toxic environments, report of the child health workgroup. April 1997. Available at: www.atsdr. cdc.gov/child/chw497.html. Accessed June 2, 2006.
[4] Etzel RA, Balk SJ. Handbook of pediatric environmental health. Elk Grove Village (IL): American Academy of Pediatrics; 1999. p. 3–4.
[5] Kirby S. Stakeholder research for marketing the PEHSU program. Presented at the PEHSU Annual Meeting. Arlington, VA; June 9, 2005.

[6] Institute of Medicine. Role of the primary care physician in occupational and environmental medicine. Washington, DC: National Academy Press; 1988. p. 1–20.

[7] Wilborne-Davis P, Kabwit MN. Enhancing the pediatric environmental health knowledge of health professionals: the role of the Pediatric Environmental Health Specialty Units (PEHSU) program, abstract and program. Presented at the American Public Health Association Annual Meeting. San Francisco, CA; November 19, 2003.

[8] Parkin R, Ragain L, Bruhl R, et al. Awwa Research Foundation. Advancing collaborations for water-related health risk communication. Denver (CO): Awwa Researcy Foundation; October 2006.

[9] Pope AM, Rall DP. Environmental medicine: integrating a missing element into medical education. Washington, DC: National Academy Press; 1995. p. 51.

[10] Etzel RA, Crain EF, Gitterman BA, et al. Pediatric environmental health competencies for specialists. Ambul Pediatr 2003;3(1):60–3.

ELSEVIER
SAUNDERS

Pediatr Clin N Am
54 (2007) 15–31

PEDIATRIC CLINICS

OF NORTH AMERICA

The Epidemiology of Pediatric Environmental Exposures

Kathryn Veal, MD, MPH[a,b,*],
Jennifer A. Lowry, MD[a,b,c],
John M. Belmont, PhD[a]

[a]*Department of Pediatrics, University of Kansas School of Medicine, 3901 Rainbow Blvd., Kansas City, KS 66160, USA*
[b]*Mid-America Pediatric Environmental Health Specialty Unit, Center for Occupational and Environmental Health, University of Kansas Medical Center, 3901 Rainbow Blvd., Kansas City, KS 66160, USA*
[c]*Mid-America Poison Control Center, University of Kansas Medical Center, 3901 Rainbow Blvd., Kansas City, KS 66160, USA*

The Agency for Toxic Substances and Disease Registry (ATSDR) estimates that 3 to 4 million children live within 1 mile of at least one hazardous waste site [1]. In addition, the US Environmental Protection Agency's (EPA) Toxics Release Inventory reports that in 2003 American industries released 4.44 billion pounds of chemical agents into the environment. Disposal or other releases of persistent bioaccumulative or toxic chemicals increased by 11% from 2002 to 2003. Disposal or other releases of lead and lead compounds increased 7% in that period, and total disposal or other releases of mercury and mercury compounds increased by 41% (although air emissions of mercury and its compounds decreased by 1%). Total disposal or other releases of dioxin and dioxinlike compounds had a net increase of 129,433 g from 2002 to 2003, but if one facility that reported an increase of 134,269 g were excluded, total disposal or other releases of dioxin and dioxinlike compounds would have decreased by 4%. Disposal or other releases of polychlorinated biphenyls increased by 20.4 million pounds from 2002 to 2003 [2].

This work was supported by funding from the Association of Occupational and Environmental Clinics, the Agency for Toxic Substances and Disease Registry, and the Environmental Protection Agency.

* Corresponding author. Department of Pediatrics, University of Kansas School of Medicine, 3901 Rainbow Blvd., Kansas City, KS 66160.

E-mail address: kveal@kumc.edu (K. Veal).

Although this information increases the understanding of the environmental exposures that children may experience, it does not help elaborate the possible health effects associated with such exposures. Epidemiologic studies have shown an increase in the incidence of asthma and cancer in children [3–8]. Although the causes of these illnesses generally are multifactorial, the influence of the child's environment cannot be discounted. Moreover, compared with adults, children may be particularly vulnerable because of developmental differences. Children are limited to their physical space and also differ from adults in their breathing capacity (eg, oxygen consumption, minute ventilation) and pharmacokinetics and pharmacodynamics (absorption, distribution, metabolism, and excretion) of the toxic chemical [9].

The difficulty in defining the health effects in children from environmental exposures also is multifactorial. First, the very definition of "environmental" is ambiguous, subjective, and, therefore, somewhat arbitrary. Second, the data to assess environmental health effects in children are largely inaccessible. There is no central database, and although the Centers for Disease Control and Prevention (CDC) has begun to implement the National Environmental Public Health tracking program, this database is in its initial stages and relies on other agencies to supply data in support of a surveillance network [10]. In addition, other private and state agencies have compiled data for environmental surveillance, but this information is largely incomplete because of differences in the target environmental sources and in the geographic areas. Although the health departments of various states do have divisions of environmental epidemiology to aid in surveillance, many of these agencies track only infectious exposures and do not evaluate other environmental health problems.

Given this general lack of information, the number of children affected by environmental exposures is unknown. Several databases, however, can be used to estimate the types of exposures of concern and where these exposures may occur. Although the CDC tracking system is incomplete, its data and the information provided in the National Report on Human Exposures to Environmental Chemicals can help in determining the environmental chemicals to which children are exposed. In addition, data from the American Association of Poison Control Centers (AAPCC) and the Pediatric Environmental Health Specialty Units (PEHSUs) may shed light on the types of exposures that are of concern to health care professionals and the general public. To support analyses reported later in this article, the authors obtained raw data from the PEHSUs (April 1, 2004 to March 31, 2005) and the AAPCC (January 1, 2004 to December 31, 2004). Of the 786 children reported to the PEHSUs in the United States during this time period, 616 child exposures were analyzed. In addition, the authors analyzed 764,949 of the 883,378 nonpharmaceutical exposures reported to the AAPCC. They did not analyze exposures to substances in categories that they did not consider environmental, such as envenomations, food poisonings, sporting equipment, and unknown substances. Although some of these numbers are large, the data sets are limited as estimates of total exposures. The bias probably is toward underreporting because the kinds and amounts of information given to the agencies depend on the individual parent's or health care worker's interests and concerns of the moment.

National epidemiologic data

No complete databases exist for pediatric exposures to the environment. In 2000, the Association of Occupational and Environmental Clinics, in cooperation with the ATSDR and EPA, established the network of PEHSUs. There is a PEHSU dedicated to each of the 10 EPA regions within the United States, and others are located in Canada and Mexico (see the map in the article by Wilborne-Davis, Kirkland, and Mulloy in this issue, page 3). The PEHSU staff in each region includes a pediatrician, an occupational/ environmental physician, and others knowledgeable about pediatric environmental exposures. The PEHSUs are meant to provide education and consultation for health professionals, public health professionals, and others concerned with children's environmental health. Each contact made to a PEHSU is documented and submitted quarterly to the national office for evaluation. Table 1 summarizes the 10 most common PEHSU categories for exposures reported between April 2004 and March 2005. These data are shown for each of the 10 EPA regions along with the national totals. Forty categories were used in the period covered, but the 10 most common accounted for 582 (94.5%) of the 616 children involved. Each substance is ranked by the number of contacts made to each regional PEHSU and overall. The most numerous calls to PEHSUs have to do with exposure to lead (36% of the 616 children), followed by fungus/mold (18%), gases/fumes (9%), mercury (8%), and indoor air contaminants (8%).

There are obvious limitations to using PEHSU data for evaluating pediatric environmental exposures. The PEHSU program is not well known, as reflected in the as-yet very small numbers of documented exposures. The cases that are documented can be classified variously within the PEHSU system, which tends to obscure the true incidence of an exposure. For example, PEHSU uses the category "gases/fumes" and also subcategories for natural gas, gases/fumes–carbon monoxide, carbon monoxide, and gases/fumes– formaldehyde. The separation or combination of such subcategories is driven by the analysts' purposes across time and agencies.

The definition of a pediatric environmental exposure can be broad enough to include all aspects of a child's environment. For that reason, the authors requested all nonpharmaceutical exposure data from the AAPCC. The AAPCC consists of 61 member poison control centers within the United States that submit their data on a real-time basis to the Toxic Exposure Surveillance System (TESS). These data are used to identify

Table 1
The 10 categories of exposures most commonly reported to Pediatric Environmental Health Specialty Units (PEHSUs) in the United States*

PEHSU category	Environmental Protection Agency Region**																				Total US	
	1		2		3		4		5		6		7		8		9		10			
	R	#	R	#	R	#	R	#	R	#	R	#	R	#	R	#	R	#	R	#	R	#
Lead	1	156	1	19	3	3	3	2	3	20	4	2	5	4	1	3	2	8	5	2	1	219
Fungus/mold	2	27	6	5	1	9	1	4	1	24	1	5	3	5	1	3	1	21	1	9	2	112
Gases/fumes	4	11	2	11	5	1	—	—	6	15	7	1	1	6	—	—	3	7	4	3	3	55
Mercury	3	13	4	6	4	2	1	4	4	16	4	2	5	4	—	—	6	1	—	—	4	48
Indoor air contaminants	6	6	8	6	2	6	6	1	4	16	4	2	5	4	6	1	6	1	2	6	4	48
Pesticides	7	4	4	2	—	—	—	—	1	24	—	—	7	1	—	—	5	2	8	1	6	35
Arsenic	5	9	8	2	—	—	—	—	7	9	2	4	—	—	—	—	4	3	—	—	7	28
Water toxins	10	1	10	1	—	—	3	3	8	8	—	—	1	6	5	2	6	1	3	4	8	23
Perchlorate	—	—	3	7	—	—	—	—	—	—	—	—	—	—	—	—	—	—	—	—	9	7
Soil toxins	—	—	7	3	—	—	—	—	—	—	—	—	—	—	—	—	—	—	5	2	9	7
Total number of children involved in top 10 categories		227		62		21		14		132		16		30		9		44		27		582

* These 10 categories account for 582 (94.5%) of the 616 children involved in calls to PEHSUs between April 1, 2004 and March 31, 2005 and included in this analysis.

** Regions are identified on the map provided by Wilborne-Davis, Kirkland, and Mulloy on page 3.

Abbreviations: R, rank; #, number of exposures reported.

Data from Wilborne-Davis P. Agency for Toxic Substances and Disease Registry (ATSDR) Quarterly Reports for PEHSU Program (through cooperative agreement U50/ATU 300014 with the Association of Occupational and Environmental Clinics). Submitted October 2005.

hazards quickly, focus prevention education, guide clinical research, direct training, and detect chemical or bioterrorism incidents. In 2004, 2,438,644 exposures were reported, of which 1,588,948 (65.2%) were in children age 19 years or younger [11]. Data from the AAPCC showed that 883,378 (55.6%) of these child exposures resulted from nonpharmaceutical substances. On reviewing these substances, the authors removed certain categories (envenomations, food poisoning, sports equipment, and unknown exposures) to reflect a more traditional definition of a child's environment. The remaining 764,949 incidents (86.6% of the total nonpharmaceutical exposures) were used to assess the most common culprits that resulted in calls to poison control centers within the United States.

Not surprisingly, the authors found that exposures in children resulted largely from products to which children had easy access. Tables 2 and 3 show the 20 most common nonpharmaceutical exposures in children reported to poison control centers. AAPCC data are supplied according to several classifications. The numbers in Table 2 relate to the AAPCC's 524 exposure substances (minor categories). Each of those substances is contained in one and only one of the 43 TESS exposure categories. The numbers in Table 3 relate to those TESS categories. The authors present both classifications here because certain substances within the TESS categories individually account for significant numbers of exposures. Of particular note, the 732,248 exposures included in the top 20 TESS categories account for more than 95% of the 764,949 exposures that the authors considered for this report.

In fact, 8 of the 20 most frequently reported substances (see Table 2) are contained in the top-ranked TESS category shown in Table 3—cosmetics/personal care products. In order of frequency these include toothpaste with fluoride, cream/lotion/make-up, perfume/cologne/aftershave, deodorant (not to be confused with deodorizers), soap (bar, hand or complexion), suntan/sunscreen products, nail polish, and peroxide. Only one household cleaning substance—bleach: hypochlorite (liquid and dry)—found a place among the top 20 substances, but it nevertheless accounts for 26,794 exposures (3.51% of 764,949 total exposures), placing it second overall. The most frequently encountered environmental exposure is desiccant (the small white pouches found in shoeboxes and other storage containers), which is joined by glow products as one of two foreign bodies/toys/miscellaneous products on the list of top 20 substances. At rank number one, desiccant accounts for 42,321 exposures (5.5% of the total exposures). Pen or ink is the fifth most common substance exposure and is the only representative of the TESS category, arts/crafts/office supply.

The most frequently encountered substances are not necessarily the most dangerous and do not necessarily account for most of the adverse medical outcomes reported. According to the authors' analysis of the AAPCC outcomes data (Table 4), ethanol (beverage), carbon monoxide, bleach: hypochlorite (liquid and dry), lamp oil, and gasoline were the top five

Table 2
The 20 nonpharmaceutical substances most commonly reported to the American Association of Poison Control Centers (AAPCC)*

AAPCC Substance	1		2		3		4		5		6		7		8		9		10		Total US	
	R	#	R	#	R	#	R	#	R	#	R	#	R	#	R	#	R	#	R	#	R	#
Desiccant	1	1613	1	3575	1	4222	1	8430	1	7315	1	5481	1	1952	1	1672	1	6207	1	1854	1	42,321
Bleach: hypochlorite (liquid and dry)	6	884	4	1745	2	2644	2	6053	2	4597	2	3902	2	1303	4	1089	2	3383	6	1194	2	26,794
Toothpaste with fluoride	2	1445	5	1579	5	2305	3	3806	3	4388	5	2175	4	1230	2	1414	3	2926	2	1560	3	22,828
Cream/lotion/make-up	3	1427	3	1827	4	2411	4	3724		—	4	2495	3	1270		112	4	2506	4	1248	4	22,324
Pen/Ink	4	1328	2	1864	3	2446	8	3008	5	3543	8	1683	8	940	8	660	6	2000	9	787	5	18,259
Perfume/cologne/aftershave	12	729	6	1210	6	1787	5	3186	6	3196	7	1871	7	964	6	743	8	1846	10	783	6	16,315
Deodorant	9	830	7	1162	7	1679	7	3103	7	3004	6	2001	6	992	7	732	9	1845	7	932	7	16,280
Soap (bar, hand or complexion)	8	831	8	1102	8	1529	9	2414	5	3220	10	1431	10	688	12	586	5	2201	12	713	8	14,715
Long-acting anticoagulant rodenticide	26	343	14	727	12	1043	6	3142	9	2844	3	2773	5	1047	5	833	14	1221	16	612	9	14,585
Plant: unknown toxic or unknown if toxic	5	926	9	951	10	1285	17	1862	10	788	13	1348	19	506	13	559	7	1864	3	1353	10	13,442
Plant: nontoxic	7	874	13	747	11	1178	11	2370		139	18	1108	13	589	9	622	13	1250	5	1214	11	12,091
Plant: gastrointestinal irritant (nonoxalate)	13	685	16	682	9	1428	12	2188	15	728	9	1479	15	552	21	414	11	1287	8	814	12	11,257
Suntan/sunscreen	11	731	11	857	13	1036	18	1732	13	805	23	868	18	517	15	546	10	1605	17	570	13	10,267
Nail polish	15	505	15	707	14	1025	19	1728	12	1028	17	1169	12	618	14	551	12	1257	14	635	14	10,223
Glow product	10	768	10	890	16	807	15	2021	16	647	15	1235	16	541	10	612	37	602	11	759	15	9882
Plant: oxalate	18	430	38	361	20	720	10	2371	16	664	19	1053	9	861	16	517	15	974	15	621	16	9572
Insect repellent with diethyltoluamide	14	660	21	499	15	833	14	2025	14	794	12	1373	11	624	11	603	49	497	50	252	17	9160

Environmental Protection Agency Region**

	R	#	R	#	R	#	R	#	R	#	R	#	R	#	R	#	R	#	R	#	R	Total
Peroxide	24	378	19	539	33	590	16	1918	18	563	11	1383	14	562	17	483	55	440	18	565	18	8421
Gasoline	41	262	50	289	18	736	13	2027	19	562	14	1333	17	537	19	424	34	684	21	503	19	8357
Ethanol (beverage)	23	384	12	757	21	718	35	1012	21	296	20	1040	21	423	28	343	16	1119	20	508	20	7600
Exposures in overall top 20 categories		16,033		22,070		30,422		58,120		56,373		37,201		16,716		14,531		35,714		17,513		304,693
Total exposures		39,969		54,629		78,416		141,739		142,483		91,810		42,449		38,558		90,405		44,491		764,949
Percentage of total represented in overall top 20		40.1%		40.4%		38.8%		41.0%		39.6%		40.5%		39.4%		37.7%		39.5%				

* Ordered by total numbers of pediatric exposures in the United States in 2004. These top 20 substances account for 39.8% of the 764,949 exposures in the United States.

** Regions are identified on the map provided by Wilborne-Davis, Kirkland, and Mulloy on page 3.

Abbreviations: R, rank; #, number of exposures reported.

Data from Watson WA, Litovitz TL, Rodgers GC Jr, et al. 2004 annual report of the American Association of Poison Control Centers Toxic Exposure Surveillance System. Am J Emerg Med 2005;23(5):589–666.

Table 3
The 20 most commonly reported Toxic Exposure Surveillance System (TESS) categories of nonpharmaceutical environmental substances*

TESS Category	Environmental Protection Agency Region**																				Total US	
	1		2		3		4		5		6		7		8		9		10			
	R	#	R	#	R	#	R	#	R	#	R	#	R	#	R	#	R	#	R	#	R	#
Cosmetics/personal care products	1	10,173	1	13,912	1	19,172	1	33,825	1	34,828	1	20,920	1	10,151	1	9234	1	22,201	1	10,329	1	184,745
Cleaning substances (household)	2	6360	2	9523	2	14,039	2	25,913	2	25,425	2	16,785	2	7807	2	7887	2	16,075	2	8002	2	137,816
Foreign bodies/toys/miscellaneous	4	3313	3	8383	3	5796	3	6809	4	13,082	3	12,066	8	3350	3	2972	3	8861	4	3425	3	68,057
Plants	3	4062	5	3362	5	3758	4	6179	5	11,538	4	11,611	4	6669	5	2884	4	7911	3	5564	4	63,538
Pesticides	6	2441	4	3823	6	3455	5	5433	3	13,523	5	11,009	2	9591	4	2926	5	5990	5	2627	5	60,818
Arts/crafts/office supplies	5	2930	6	1511	4	4196	6	5011	6	6273	6	7381	6	3654	6	1961	6	4287	6	1844	6	39,048
Alcohols	7	1267	7	1372	7	2202	7	2791	8	5021	7	5167	5	3699	7	1541	7	3901	7	1526	7	28,487
Hydrocarbons	9	1011	8	1265	9	1189	8	2369	7	5112	8	4560	7	3360	8	1442	8	2720	8	1479	8	24,507
Deodorizers	11	858	9	929	10	1167	9	2201	9	4169	9	3892	10	2687	9	1238	10	1961	9	1127	9	20,229
Chemicals	8	1013	12	736	8	1371	10	1869	10	3009	11	3122	9	2790	10	842	9	2169	10	965	10	17,886
Paints and stripping agents	10	947	11	830	11	1141	11	1623	11	2329	12	2698	11	1399	12	750	11	1860	11	859	11	14,436
Fumes/gases/vapors	12	640	10	875	12	893	12	1471	13	1831	10	3174	13	1197	11	786	12	1374	14	569	12	12,810
Adhesives and glues	13	611	13	601	13	742	13	1194	12	1988	13	2064	12	1329	13	656	13	1319	13	618	13	11,122
Polishes and waxes	17	403	15	480	14	503	15	895	14	1465	14	1534	14	1059	15	518	17	968	17	451	14	8276

Category	Rank	Region 1 # (R)	Region 2 # (R)	Region 3 # (R)	Region 4 # (R)	Region 5 # (R)	Region 6 # (R)	Region 7 # (R)	Region 8 # (R)	Region 9 # (R)	Region 10 # (R)	Total
Batteries	16	404 (14)	622 (15)	761 (16)	1382 (15)	1389 (15)	908 (16)	395 (18)	359 (16)	917 (18)	416 (15)	7553
Fertilizers	14	435 (19)	369 (19)	598 (17)	1170 (16)	1377 (17)	733 (18)	332 (14)	504 (17)	825 (15)	546 (16)	6939
Tobacco products	20	361 (21)	348 (16)	720 (18)	1155 (17)	1426 (16)	864 (15)	492 (24)	274 (19)	696 (16)	521 (17)	6857
Mushrooms	18	402 (22)	335 (23)	496 (19)	1076 (19)	1179 (19)	710 (23)	338 (16)	427 (14)	972 (12)	786 (18)	6691
Swimming pool/aquarium supplies	21	290 (18)	431 (17)	718 (14)	1509 (20)	1207 (18)	729 (17)	391 (23)	286 (18)	791 (23)	326 (19)	6678
Building/construction material	15	412 (17)	448 (20)	596 (23)	826 (21)	1189 (23)	558 (21)	325 (19)	327 (20)	691 (20)	383 (20)	5755
Total exposures in top 20 categories		38,333	52,401	74,945	136,196	136,298	88,024	40,520	36,679	86,489	42,363	732,248
Total exposures		39,969	54,629	78,416	141,739	142,483	91,810	42,449	38,558	90,405	44,491	764,949
Percentage of total represented in top 20		95.9%	95.9%	95.6%	96.1%	95.7%	95.9%	95.5%	95.1%	95.7%	95.2%	95.7%

* Ordered by total pediatric exposures in the United States in 2004. These 20 categories account for 95.7% of the 764,949 exposures in the United States.

** Regions are identified on the map provided by Wilborne-Davis, Kirkland, and Mulloy on page 3.

Abbreviations: R, rank; #, number of exposures reported.

Data from Watson WA, Litovitz TL, Rodgers GC Jr, et al. 2004 annual report of the American Association of Poison Control Centers Toxic Exposure Surveillance System. Am J Emerg Med 2005;23(5):589–666.

Table 4
The 20 most dangerous nonpharmaceutical environmental substances*

Substance	TESS Category	Outcome			
		Death	Major	Moderate	Overall
Ethanol (beverage)	Alcohols	2	54	476	532
Carbon monoxide	Fumes/gases/vapors	8	22	151	181
Bleach: hypochlorite (liquid & dry)	Cleaning substances (household)	—	4	149	153
Mushroom: hallucinogenic	Mushrooms	—	3	112	115
Lamp oil	Hydrocarbons	—	7	100	107
Gasoline	Hydrocarbons	—	5	76	81
Plant: anticholinergic	Plants	—	9	58	67
Wall/floor/tile/all-purpose cleaner: alkali	Cleaning substances (household)	—	2	64	66
Freon/other propellant	Fumes/gases/vapors	—	5	56	61
Unknown mushroom	Mushrooms	—	2	57	59
Chlorine gas	Fumes/gases/vapors	—	3	50	53
Other acid	Chemicals	—	3	46	49
Cyanoacrylate	Adhesives and glues	—	—	49	49
Alkali (excluding cleaners, bleach, etc.)	Chemicals	—	3	45	48
Pyrethroid	Pesticides	—	1	46	47
Other hydrocarbon	Hydrocarbons	—	1	45	46
Miscellaneous cleaning agents: alkali	Cleaning substances (household)	—	1	44	45
Penlight/flashlight/dry cell battery	Batteries	—	—	45	45
Industrial cleaner: alkali	Industrial cleaners	—	3	38	41
Ammonia (excluding cleaners)	Chemicals	—	2	38	40

* Based on numbers of deaths and major and moderate outcomes of children's exposures to them. These 20 substances account for 44.8% of the 4205 significant outcomes reported for 2004.

Abbreviation: TESS, Toxic Exposure Surveillance System.

Data from Watson WA, Litovitz TL, Rodgers GC Jr, et al. 2004 annual report of the American Association of Poison Control Centers Toxic Exposure Surveillance System. Am J Emerg Med 2005;23(5):589–666.

exposures that resulted in moderate and major outcomes including death. A moderate outcome is one in which the patient exhibits signs or symptoms requiring some sort of treatment. A major outcome is one in which the patient has a life-threatening event or has a disability as a result of the exposure [11]. One substance commonly recognized as toxic is alkaline industrial cleaner, ingestions of which are often referred for endoscopy because of its high potential for significant morbidity or death [12]. Alkaline industrial cleaner is not included in the top 20 substances reported to the poison control centers, however. Instead, the household cleaner that ranks as number two for common exposures substances and also is the third most common substance with major or moderate outcomes is bleach: hypochlorite.

Plants account for 4 of the 20 top substance exposures reported to AAPCC. Most common are those that are unknown to the caller (the child was unable to identify the plant) or whose toxicity is unknown. These are followed by plants that are known to be nontoxic. The most commonly reported specifically identified plants are non-oxalate gastrointestinal irritants (eg, daffodils, *Narcissus pseudonarcissus*) and oxalates (eg, *Philodendron* spp) The relative toxicity of most household and yard or garden plants is unknown or is variously under- or overappreciated by most parents.

Gasoline, a hydrocarbon, and ethanol beverages (alcohol) round out the top-20 list of pediatric environmental exposures for 2004. Although each category has only one representative on the list, these products, like hypochlorite bleach, comprise enough exposures to put the entire category on the list of TESS top 10 categories (see Table 3). Conversely, the categories of deodorizers, chemicals, paints and stripping agents, and fumes/gases/ vapors have no representative substances on the list of top 20 exposures (see Table 2).

One must appreciate certain limitations in the AAPCC data sets. First and foremost, the information is limited to that actually reported to each participating center by the public. The data, therefore, are best regarded as supporting an epidemiology of poison exposures that cause enough concern to warrant a telephone call by a knowledgeable caller. In addition, the AAPCC data are not readily accessible to public health agencies or other health care professionals who may be interested in the prevalence of exposures in a particular geographical area. Although the real-time surveillance system allows agencies to be aware of what may be occurring in their communities, the published documents largely include only national data and do not allow for a more refined epidemiologic database, hence, more refined analyses.

In addition to the databases addressing the concerns of the public and health care professionals, the CDC recently released its Third National Report on Human Exposure to Environmental Chemicals [13]. Based on biomonitoring, this document reports on the most recent assessment of exposures to environmental chemicals in the United States. It reports on 148 environmental chemicals or their metabolites in blood and urine from a random sample of participants from the National Health and Nutrition Examination Survey. Although these data do not focus on the concerns of the public regarding environmental exposures, they do provide estimates of actual exposures to certain substances for the United States population.

Of particular note, the authors found that none of the chemicals tested for by the CDC are addressed in the 20 exposures most commonly called in to United States poison control centers. The 2005 CDC report recently added the pyrethroid insecticides (number 21 of AAPCC data) to those that are assessed in the United States population. This is the first time this chemical has been listed, and reference values are not yet available. The findings, however, suggest a widespread exposure to the chemicals for which the CDC tested. Currently, there is little information about the health effects from these exposures.

In contrast, the CDC document does comment on some environmental exposures that are reported to PEHSUs. Notably, there are data on progress in eliminating lead from children. For the period from 1999 to 2002, 1.6% of children aged 1 to 5 years had elevated blood lead levels. This percentage is a solid decrease from the 4.4% reported for the early 1990s. In addition, in the period from 1999 to 2002, no women of childbearing age had levels at or above that associated with neurodevelopmental effects on the fetus. Exposures to other heavy metals and pesticides are assessed and encompass the majority of exposures documented in the CDC report. Thus, the report is an informative reference on which chemicals get into Americans and at what concentrations. Trends, over time, can be determined, and research can be guided by these data. The report documents only exposures to these chemicals, however, and cannot address the toxicity or ultimately, the health effects for the majority of them. The information simply is not known.

These databases, despite their limitations, provide the information available for the pediatrician and other health care professionals to use to determine what types of environmental exposures are important to the families they serve. Educating health care providers and the public regarding these exposures can aid in their proper diagnosis and treatment, and reassurance can be given confidently more often.

Regional epidemiologic data

The EPA divides the United States into 10 administrative regions, each including specific states (see the map in the article by Wilborne-Davis, Kirkland, and Mulloy in this issue, page 3). Thus, each EPA region may have unique characteristics that may predispose children to particular exposures. General characteristics for each region are included in Table 5. Although the populations in different regions vary, the percentage of children under the age of 18 years is uniform across all regions, at about 25%. Differences occur in the percentage of the population living in rural areas. The US Census Bureau classifies an urban area as all territory, population, and housing units that have census blocks with a density of at least 1000 people per square mile at the time, surrounded by blocks that have at least 500 people per square mile. Rural areas consist of all territory, population, and housing units located outside these urban areas [14]. Specifically, regions with more rural areas (eg, regions 4 and 7) may be predisposed to exposures related to agriculture or outdoor contaminants. Regions with more urban areas (eg, regions 2 and 9) may have a higher percentage of indoor or urban exposures.

The Superfund program was established in 1980 to locate, investigate, and clean up the most contaminated sites nationwide. The EPA administers the Superfund program in cooperation with individual states and tribal governments. The National Priorities List is the list of national priorities among the known releases or threatened releases of hazardous substances,

Table 5
Demographics and releases of toxics in each Environmental Protection Agency region and the total for the United States*

	Environmental Protection Agency region**										Total US
	1	2	3	4	5	6	7	8	9	10	
Total population (in millions)	13.9	31.2	27.8	53.3	50.1	33.3	12.9	9.3	42.2	11.2	285.2
Child population (in millions)	3.4	7.9	6.7	13.1	13.0	9.2	3.3	2.5	11.4	2.9	73.4
Child population (%)	24.2	25.2	24.2	24.6	25.9	27.6	25.7	27.3	27.1	26.0	25.7
Rural population (in millions)	2.5	3.1	6.6	16.1	11.5	7.8	4.1	2.2	2.8	2.4	59.0
Rural population (%)	17.6	9.8	23.7	30.3	23.0	23.4	32.0	23.2	6.5	21.7	20.7
Number of sites on the Final National Priorities List	184	225	176	174	250	90	126	78	140	141	1584
Total Toxics Release Inventory (million lbs)	30.9	76.0	402.5	883.4	803.7	483.2	220.4	363.4	512.6	665.5	4441.6
Toxics (in lbs) released per child	9	10	60	68	62	53	66	143	45	228	61

* "Rural" and "child" are defined in the text. The Final National Priorities List targets specific toxic substances. The Toxics Release Inventory reports amounts of substances released.

** Regions are identified on the map provided by Wilborne-Davis, Kirkland, and Mulloy on page 3.

Data from US Census Bureau. US census data 2000. Available at: http://www.census.gov. Accessed March 30, 2006.

pollutants, or contaminants in the Superfund program. The Toxics Release Inventory is an annual EPA report on toxic chemical releases and other waste-management activities. The report comments on the number of pounds of specific chemicals released by these facilities. The number of sites on or part of a final National Priorities List and the number of pounds (in millions) for each region is included in Table 5.

Summary of findings

After taking into account the limitations of the databases, it still may be possible to glean broad impressions of regional similarities and distinctions. Calls to the PEHSUs are made by parents, physicians, health department workers, and federal agency officials among others. They tend to focus on exposures that are more overtly environmental in nature and often involve multiple children, whereas calls to the poison control centers tend to relate to a single child who has ingested a substance. The differences between the substances noted in Tables 1 and 2 reflect this variance in focus.

The PEHSUs receive markedly fewer calls than the poison control centers. There were 1003 total PEHSU contacts during the 12 months included in Table 1; 636 were exposure contacts, and 367 were information contacts. Caller concerns ranged from the nonspecific ("something in the house" believed to be responsible for symptoms a child is experiencing) to the well documented (notification by ATSDR of a geographically specific toxic spill). Because of the smaller number of calls, there is less variation in numbers of exposures between categories. Therefore, in many instances, the "rankings" of substances of concern are not informative. For example, although "gases/ fumes" holds rank number one in Region 7, there were only one or two more exposures in this category than in the others ranked.

In certain PEHSUs call data are skewed toward certain substances because of an announced topic of concern. For example, the Region 1 PEHSU, located at Boston Children's Hospital, offers a Lead Clinic, resulting in a high percentage (70%) of PEHSU exposures related to lead. Lead, however, is an issue for PEHSUs across the country. Only Regions 6 and 10 fail to document lead as one of the top three substances of concern for the year. If the lead exposures in Region 1 were reduced to reflect their relatively reduced importance across the remaining regions, the estimate for Region 1 would drop lead exposures to rank number two.

There are additional examples of regional skewing. Fungus/mold exposures, at overall rank number two, accounted for 15% of the PEHSU total. This category is ranked first or second except in Region 2, where it ranks sixth. Additionally, without further information, one can only speculate why so many more pesticide exposures were reported to the Region 5 PEHSU than in other highly agricultural regions. For these reasons, the authors concentrate on the more generally applicable exposure data from the AAPCC to illustrate regional similarities and distinctions.

The AAPCC data for 2004 summarized in Table 3 are arranged in order of occurrence by TESS category. These categories consolidate product substances into what can be characterized loosely as usage groups. The frequency of pediatric exposure to products within these groups probably results from their abundance and accessibility within children's home environments. Cosmetics and personal care products, household cleaning substances, arts and crafts and office supplies, and deodorizers often are easily accessible. Most of these products are seemingly innocuous and may not be included in parental efforts to protect children from toxic exposure by keeping dangerous items behind locked cabinet doors. Items within the foreign bodies category include children's toys, such as glow products and bubble-blowing solution, as well as elements of daily living such as soil and glass. Household plants and common yard plantings of varying toxicity are frequent offenders. Included among pesticide exposures are products specifically applied to children's bodies to eradicate lice and protect against the bites of insects that might carry West Nile virus and other infectious entities. These include pyrethroids, insect repellents with diethyltoluamide (DEET), and those without DEET.

Ranking of these exposures is highly uniform across the country, with cosmetics/personal care products and household cleaning substances rated first and second, respectively, in every region. The category of foreign bodies/toys/miscellaneous ranks third or fourth in all regions except Region 7, in which pesticide exposures rank third. Pesticides are also third in Region 4. All regions rank plants as third, fourth, or fifth, generally followed by pesticides. Arts/crafts/office supplies are ranked sixth in 7 of the 10 regions, occurring more frequently in Regions 1 and 2 and slightly less frequently in Region 6. Alcohols, including ethanol (beverage and nonbeverage) as well as isopropanol, methanol, and various rubbing alcohols, are at rank number seven in 8 of the 10 regions—slightly higher in Region 6 (number six) and slightly lower in Region 4 (number 8). Hydrocarbons (gasoline, lubricating and motor oils, lamp oil and kerosene, lighter fluid, mineral spirits), deodorizers (air fresheners, toilet bowl and diaper pail deodorizers), and various chemicals (noncleaning ammonias, alkalis, and acids, nonmedicinal nitrates and nitrites, nonautomotive glycols, formaldehyde and formalin) round out the top 10 categories in most regions. Paints and stripping agents is the final category on the list in Region 1, with fumes/gases/vapors (carbon monoxide and dioxide, methane and natural gas, hydrogen sulfide or sewer gas, propane, chlorine and chloramine) listed as number 10 in Regions 5 and 8.

Summary

Despite the limitations of their current databases for research, the PEHSU and poison control centers remain the best resource for the general public and for health care professionals who have questions regarding pediatric environmental health. Both agencies are staffed by professionals who have been trained in poisonings and have expertise in environmental toxicology.

According to the Institute of Medicine, there have been advances in the research fields of environmental health, particularly concerning hazards to human health that may result from environmental exposures. It is known that air pollution can cause respiratory disease, and heavy metals can cause neurotoxicity [15]. The 1997 Executive Order 13045–Protection of Children From Environmental Health Risks and Safety Risks stated that each federal agency should make it a high priority to identify and assess risks posed to children by the environment. Many programs were instituted at that time to help assess the epidemiology of pediatric environmental health. These programs included the Voluntary Children's Chemical Evaluation Program, the Children's Environmental Health and Safety Inventory of Research, and the National Children's Study. Only the National Children's Study is ongoing, but it may end prematurely because of cuts in federal funding.

Currently, the only national databases that are available to aid in a search to assess the effect of environmental exposures on children's health are those provided by the PEHSUs and the poison control centers. Both have limitations and are largely deficient in accurate, helpful numbers. Both, however, offer insight into factors that are important to the public and health care professionals and provide some outcome data to measure morbidity and mortality. The CDC has begun to offer insight on what factors should be important to the public and health care professionals. One hopes that the two sets of data will converge in the future as the PEHSUs become better known and more widely used and as coding and analysis schemes are harmonized across programs.

References

[1] Agency for Toxic Substances and Disease Registry (US). Children's health. Available at: http://www.atsdr.cdc.gov/child/ochchildhlth.html. Accessed February 28, 2006.
[2] U.S. Environmental Protection Agency. 2003 TRI public data release brochure. Washington, DC: Environmental Protection Agency; 2005.
[3] Knorr RS, Condon SK, Dwyer FM, et al. Tracking pediatric asthma: the Massachusetts experience using school health records. Environ Health Perspect 2004;112:1424–7.
[4] Delfino RJ. Epidemiologic evidence for asthma and exposure to air toxics: linkages between occupational, indoor, and community air pollution research. Environ Health Perspect 2002; 110(Suppl 4):573–89.
[5] Johnson CC, Ownby DR, Zoratti EM, et al. Environmental epidemiology of pediatric asthma and allergy. Epidemiol Rev 2002;24:154–75.
[6] Etzel RA. How environmental exposures influence the development and exacerbation of asthma. Pediatrics 2003;112:233–9.
[7] Daniels JL, Olshan AF, Teschke K, et al. Residential pesticide exposure and neuroblastoma. Epidemiology 2001;12:20–7.

[8] Linet MS, Wacholder S, Zahm SH. Interpreting epidemiologic research: lessons from studies on childhood cancer. Pediatrics 2003;112:218–32.

[9] Kearns GL, Abdel-Rahman SM, Alander SW, et al. Developmental pharmacology: drug disposition, action, and therapy in infants and children. N Engl J Med 2003;349: 1157–67.

[10] Centers for Disease Control and Prevention (US). National environmental public health tracking program. Available at: http://www.cdc.gov/nceh/tracking. Accessed March 30, 2006.

[11] Watcon WA, Litovitz TL, Rodgers GC Jr, et al. 2004 annual report of the American Association of Poison Control Centers Toxic Exposure Surveillance System. Am J Emerg Med 2005;23(5):589–666.

[12] Poley JW, Steyerberg EW, Kuipers EJ, et al. Ingestion of acid and alkaline agents: outcome and prognostic value of early upper endoscopy. Gastrointest Endosc 2004;60:372–7.

[13] Centers for Disease Control and Prevention. Third national report on human exposure to environmental chemicals. Washington, DC: Department of Health and Human Services; 2005.

[14] US Census Bureau. US census data 2000. Available at: http://www.census.gov. Accessed March 30, 2006.

[15] Hanna K, Coussens C. Rebuilding the unity of health and the environment: a new vision of environmental health for the 21st century. Washington, DC: The National Academies Press; 2001. p. 2.

ELSEVIER
SAUNDERS

Pediatr Clin N Am
54 (2007) 33–46

PEDIATRIC CLINICS

OF NORTH AMERICA

Effective Risk Communication in Children's Environmental Health: Lessons Learned from 9/11

Maida P. Galvez, MD, MPH[a],*,
Richard Peters, DrPH, MBA, MSc[b],
Nathan Graber, MD, MPH[a], Joel Forman, MD[a]

[a]Mount Sinai School of Medicine, 1 Gustave L. Levy Place,
Box 1512, New York, NY 10029, USA
[b]Center for Risk Communication, 29 Washington Square West,
Suite 2, New York, NY 10011, USA

"… the major public health challenges since 9/11 were not just clinical, epidemiological, technical, issues. The major challenges were communication. In fact, as we move into the 21st century, communication may well become the central science of public health practice."

Edward Baker, MD, MPH
Assistant US Surgeon General
December 2001

The importance of effective risk communication

In situations with real and visible threats to the health of children, such as the World Trade Center disaster on September 11, 2001 (9/11), pediatric health care providers must be prepared to communicate the health risks of environmental exposures in childhood. In most circumstances for the pediatric provider, communication about risk typically is confined to discussions of (1) prognosis of childhood disease or disability and (2) risks and benefits of medical interventions. Discussion of health hazards related to environmental exposure differs in key ways, because the individual providing the information may not be regarded as a reliable source, topics may be unfamiliar to both the physician and the parent or guardian, and there is limited research specifically assessing risks of exposure in childhood [1].

* Corresponding author.
E-mail address: maida.galvez@mssm.edu (M.P. Galvez).

0031-3955/07/$ - see front matter © 2007 Elsevier Inc. All rights reserved.
doi:10.1016/j.pcl.2006.11.003 *pediatric.theclinics.com*

Parents often turn to the child's pediatrician with questions about environmental exposures. In a 2002 survey of health care practices affected by 9/11, pediatricians reported that although they responded to numerous questions related to 9/11, they lacked both the training and preparedness to address environmentally related health questions (Y. Yung and D. Laraque, personal communication, 2006). This finding is not surprising, because about one in four medical schools offers no instruction at all in this area, and in the schools that do the mean number of hours of instruction over 4 years of study is less than 10 hours [2]. The inability to convey information about the risk to health arising from exposure to environmental hazards is compounded by the lack of scientific information concerning the more than 80,000 synthetic chemicals produced in the United States since 1950, most of which have not been studied for their developmental toxicity to children [3]. As a consequence, the information parents obtain about environmental exposures is likely to come from sources other than their pediatric provider and may include government agencies, mass media, or websites.

This article describes the theory behind effective communication about risk using illustrative examples from the events that followed the World Trade Center disaster. It discusses in detail the experience of risk communication after 9/11, using outdoor air quality and particulate matter as examples. The authors share key lessons learned and provide a template for communicating risk, which can serve as a guide to developing a public health message for pediatric providers.

Basic principles of risk communication

The practice of risk communication is built on three basic theoretical models: risk perception, trust determination, and cognitive attenuation. These models provide insight into the ways in which an audience forms perceptions about risk, establishes trust, processes information, and ultimately makes decisions about risks. They are evidence based and offer practical tools for health care providers, health educators, and public health officials, all of whom frequently are in the position of communicating information about health risks. Each of the models is discussed in this article [4,5].

Risk perception

A number of factors have been identified that affect how risks are perceived [4,6–8]. Some of the factors influencing the perception of risk are presented in Table 1. As an illustration, consider the parent who is concerned about a child's ongoing exposure to air pollution from the 9/11 disaster. Simply providing parents with direct actions they can take to control their child's exposure to airborne pollutants (eg, cleaning air conditioner filters, damp-mopping hard surfaces, and avoiding exposure to cigarette smoke)

Table 1
Factors affecting the perception of risk

Factor	Risks perceived to be...		Risks perceived to be...
Control	under an individual's control	Are more accepted than	under control of others
Familiarity	familiar		strange
Trust	associated with a trusted source		associated with an untrusted source
Certainty	known to science		unknown to science
Reversibility	reversible		irreversible
Voluntariness	voluntary		imposed
Origin	natural		generated by humans
Fairness	distributed equally		distributed unevenly
Victim's age	affecting adults		affecting children
Dread	associated with less dreaded outcomes		associated with highly dreaded outcomes

will lower the parents' perceptions of the risk of the exposure by giving them sense of control over the situation. The pediatric provider also can reduce the perceived risk of this exposure by making it more familiar and less strange or alien. This is accomplished by substituting common, everyday words for technical terms when discussing a child's exposure to an airborne pollutant (eg, substituting the words "dust, soot, and smoke" for "particulate matter"). Although effective communication cannot impact all the factors influencing risk perception, an understanding of the qualities that drive the perception of risk provides the communicator with effective tools to determine levels of concern, anxiety, and fear in a given situation. The pediatric provider can use this knowledge to formulate messages that bring the perceived degree of risk closer to reality. In the days and weeks following 9/11, the public was exposed to a variety of pollutants in airborne particulate matter. At the time of the exposure there was much scientific uncertainty and concern about irreversible and dreaded potential health outcomes, such as cancer. These factors, which tend to heighten the public's perception of risk, were outside the influence of both the general public and the person communicating the risk (often a health care provider or a public health official). As mentioned previously, however, the persons involved in risk communication were in a position to decrease the public's perception of risk by emphasizing the actions that the public could take to control exposure to the risk (eg, avoiding outdoor activities on days with poor air quality) and using familiar terminology (eg, "soot" instead of "carbon compounds").

Pediatric providers frequently use comparisons of risk in their discussions with patients and parents. Understanding the factors that influence the perception of risk can help the risk communicator avoid a common error in risk comparisons. Attempts to compare two risks with different risk perception profiles in an effort to make the risk more familiar frequently result in audience rejection of the comparison, hostility toward the communicator, and a breakdown in communication. An example of this situation is comparing the risk of dying in an earthquake in California with that of dying in another terrorist attack like 9/11, a comparison of a familiar, natural, evenly distributed risk affecting all members of the population equally with a risk that is strange, generated by humans, and unevenly distributed among a small portion of the population.

In the aftermath of 9/11, successful comparisons of air quality were made to historical background levels. Other generally accepted comparisons can be made to state and federal health-based standards, or, in their absence, to historical background levels. Although the latter address the risk indirectly, they provide a valuable frame of reference for the public.

Trust determination

A consistent theme in the literature concerning risk communication is the need to build trust [9–12]. When trust is present, perceptions of risk are lowered; when trust is absent, perceptions of risk are heightened. Building trust is integral to communicating risk effectively [4].

Four factors have been identified as key determinants of trust: the perception of (1) care and empathy; (2) honesty and openness; (3) dedication and commitment; and (4) competence and expertise [10]. Empathy is a particularly important part of communications regarding health risks [13]. As Will Rogers pointed out, "When people are upset, they want to know that you care...before they care what you know." Moreover, it has been shown that perceptions of care and empathy are the strongest factors for creating trust when people are highly concerned, anxious, or fearful [14,15].

Pediatric providers can enhance patients' perceptions of care and empathy in several ways, including active listening (eg, providing feedback and paraphrasing), mirroring (eg, identifying underlying similarities between the pediatric provider and the audience such as marital status; children, if any; and similar personal details), and removing physical barriers (eg, crossed arms, desks, podiums). The last is of particular importance because nonverbal communications often convey more than do spoken words.

When possible, it is best to choose a communicator who resides in the community. Even so, there frequently are differences in race, culture, education, and economic status. A communicator, regardless of his or her background, may highlight other points of commonality, such as parenthood, thus bridging the gaps between the communicator and the audience.

Health care providers generally are perceived as caring, honest, dedicated experts, and they have emerged as one of the most trusted and credible sources of information about environmental health risks [15]. Yet, when perceptions of risk are elevated and people are highly concerned, anxious, or fearful, the need to build trust may still exist, and simple displays of care and empathy can facilitate effective communication.

Cognitive attenuation

Research has shown that individuals experiencing high levels of concern, anxiety, or fear, whether caused by real or perceived threats, demonstrate diminished ability to process information [5]. Cognitive attenuation, also known as mental noise, can restrict communication severely. Pediatric providers may experience this situation when presenting bad news to patients or their parents. Bad news elevates concern, anxiety, and fear, resulting in limited ability to process or retain information. When mental noise is present, a narrow window exists for communicating information to individuals who are highly concerned, anxious, or fearful [16]. Measures to overcome mental noise in situations of high concern are discussed in the next section on developing a message for communicating risk.

Developing a message for communicating risk

Several rules have been developed to facilitate more effective discussions communicating risk. The first is the rule of three, based on research in cognitive load theory, which finds that people can process only two or three items of information at a time [17]. In practical terms, people have a strong ability to recall triplets. This pattern is displayed in many areas, including sporting events ("three strikes and you're out"), nursery rhymes ("three blind mice"), memorable phrases ("life, liberty, and the pursuit of happiness") and even medical symptoms, which are often grouped in three's (eg, Cushing's triad and Virchow's triad). Applying this rule dictates that communications be limited to three key messages. Further, each key message should be supported by only three facts, each supported by a further three facts. In this way, an information pyramid can be built that will enable a pediatric provider to present information that is accessible to the audience.

The second is the rule of negative amplification. This rule is based on the research finding that people accept risks associated with gain and avoid those associated with loss [18]. In addition, when facing a loss, persons give greater weight to negative information. For example, most patients would be more likely to choose a surgical procedure with a 95% success rate than one with a 5% failure rate. This finding has several implications. One is that negative information should be balanced by a larger amount of positive information. Another is that statements containing negatives (no, not, never, nothing, none) receive greater listener attention and should be avoided. Lastly, the framing of risk information can influence the acceptability of risk and ultimately the decisions a family makes regarding risk.

The third rule is to keep the message short and simple. Responses to questions are best kept to 2 minutes or less. This technique has several advantages. It helps avoid complex, possibly confusing responses; it offers increased opportunities to determine audience understanding; and it allows the time needed for listening. Clear, simple, straightforward language should be used when addressing highly concerned, anxious, or fearful adults. Language three grade levels below that attained by the adult, determined by vocabulary, sentence length, and construction, often is most successful. Because most adults have, at the minimum, a high school education, language at the ninth grade level often is suitable. When addressing audiences with less education, a lower grade level would be appropriate. To improve clarity, it is necessary to define terms plainly and to avoid acronyms (such as "CBC" for "complete blood count") and jargon (such as the use of the term "acute asthma exacerbation" instead of "asthma attack"). Although these restrictions may be lifted when speaking with medical or other professionals, retention often is enhanced when these rules are followed. For all audiences, the use of visual materials (including pictures, drawings, and graphs) greatly increases comprehension and understanding.

This section has discussed broadly the theoretical foundations of risk communications about risk and has provided some simple guidelines for their application (Fig. 1). In advance of an actual event, such as a terrorist attack, hurricane, or flood, professionals and public health officials often need to (1) identify potential issues; (2) prepare messages; and (3) identify spokespersons and credible subject matter experts in relevant fields (eg,

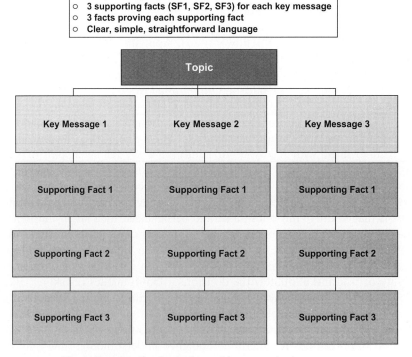

Fig. 1. Template for developing a risk communication message.

risk communication, pediatrics, toxicology, epidemiology, and public health) and train them in applying the tools and techniques of communicating about risk, a few of which have been presented here. There also is a need to select the best means for conveying information, recognizing that face-to-face dialogue is optimal when communicating risk. For further information on principles for communicating about risk and practice, please refer to Box 1.

Case study on risk communication in the aftermath of the World Trade Center disaster

In the aftermath of 9/11, environmental pollutants were evident at businesses, schools, homes, places of worship, public areas, parks, and playgrounds located in the lower Manhattan area. The population was in a state of shock and fear, which presented a significant challenge to communication

---

Box 1. Resources

Agency for Toxic Substances Disease Registry: A Primer on Health Risk Communication Principles and Practices
www.atsdr.cdc.gov/HEC/primer.html

Agency for Toxic Substances Disease Registry: ToxFAQs
http://www.atsdr.cdc.gov/toxfaq.html

American Academy of Pediatrics Committee on Environmental Health. Etzel, RA, ed. Pediatric Environmental Health "The Green Book." 2nd edition. Elk Grove Village (IL): American Academy of Pediatrics; 2003

Association of Occupational and Environmental Clinics- Pediatric Environmental Health Specialty Units (PEHSU)
http://www.aoec.org/PEHSU.htm

Centers for Disease Control: Emergency Risk Information
www.cdc.gov/communication/emergency/features/f001.htm

Center for Risk Communication
http://www.centerforriskcommunication.com/home.htm

Environmental Health From Global to Local. Frumkin H, editor. San Francisco (CA): John Wiley and Sons; 2005.

Environmental Protection Agency: Considerations in Risk Communication: A Digest of Risk Communication as a Risk Management Tool (Revised)
http://www.epa.gov/ORD/NRMRL/pubs/625r02004/625r02004.pdf

about risk. Public officials and individual physicians were faced with urgent inquiries about the health risks of the environmental exposures in lower Manhattan. Assistance was sought from many directions including the Pediatric Environmental Health Specialty Unit (PEHSU) in New York City, a resource that provides consultations for children who have toxic environmental exposures and diseases of suspected environmental origin. Parents calling the PEHSU asked whether it was safe to return home, what cleanup was recommended, and whether these exposures caused a child's asthma. Expectant mothers asked about the health of their unborn babies. Pediatricians called asking whether to expect long-term health effects related to these exposures. Schools asked when it was safe for students to return.

The situation after 9/11 presented a number of challenges to communication about risk. Many factors increased the public's perception of risk: the situation was beyond the individual's control, was unfamiliar to Americans, was imposed maliciously on the city by humans, and involved potential serious health effects resulting from environmental exposures about which the science was uncertain at best. The first communicators of information and risk were government officials who were not always physicians. Because government officials usually do not carry a high level of trust, their prominent position as communicators about risk often increased the public's perception of risk. Further, the public was faced with a barrage of often conflicting, technical, and complicated information that, given the extraordinarily high level of concern present after 9/11, was beyond its ability to process, assimilate, and retain.

To deal with these challenges, risk communicators used a number of strategies with varying degrees of effectiveness. One of the most important approaches was to present specific steps that members of the public could take to assert some level of control in their lives and reduce their exposure to potential environmental hazards, particularly dust, soot, and smoke in the air. The New York City Department of Health, the PEHSU, and the Environmental Protection Agency (EPA), among others, rapidly produced and distributed specific guidance using lay terminology. They provided advice on reducing exposures when airborne particulate matter levels were high (eg, avoiding vigorous outdoor exercise, keeping windows closed, and replacing filters on air conditioners), thus giving the public a level of personal control and reducing both anxiety and the perception of risk. This information was distributed through the media, in print, and on the Internet.

A major difficulty in assessing environmental risks to children is the large gap in knowledge regarding exposure limits for children ages 0 to 18 years and in utero. Current acceptable threshold levels for many environmental exposures are based on healthy adults in the workplace setting and do not take into account vulnerable populations with unique susceptibilities to environmental exposures, including children, the elderly, and those who have chronic health conditions (eg, heart disease and asthma).

In the aftermath of 9/11, successful comparisons of air quality were made to historical background levels. Other generally accepted comparisons were made to state and federal standards or, in the absence of such standards, to concurrent background levels. This method proved useful for comparison of both dose and duration of exposure. Although this information provided limited information on the potential for long-term health consequences of exposure, it did establish an effective and adequate frame of reference. When the magnitude of the exposure is in concordance with either current or historical background levels and is of brief duration, this sort of comparison can provide reassurance to families in the absence of evidence-based reference values or health-based exposure standards.

This general approach was employed successfully for 9/11-related exposures such as volatile organic compounds (commonly referred to as solvents), dioxins (byproducts of combustion), polychlorinated biphenyls (chlorinated hydrocarbon compounds used as coolants and lubricants), and even for toxins with existing reference ranges for sensitive populations, such as lead. For example, both the collapse of the World Trade Center and the continued fires at the site led to the release of particulate matter, microscopic particles referred to as "PM2.5" and "PM10" based on the size of the particles. Particulate matter is a major indicator of outdoor air quality, and several regulatory agencies, including the EPA, monitor levels in the air on a continuous basis in urban, suburban, and rural areas. EPA data indicate that in the immediate aftermath of 9/11 there were large increases in short-term levels of PM2.5 at and above the Air Quality Index level of 40 $\mu g/m^3$. In general, these elevations of particulate matter levels followed the path of the smoke plumes, depending on wind direction. Levels of particulate matter were higher at night, in part because of changes in temperature and air movement, and were lower on rainy days because the rain washed some of the particulate matter from the air. Although some hourly levels as high as 200 $\mu g/m^3$ were reported, 24-hour averages for these same areas were significantly lower, at 40 to 90 $\mu g/m^3$.

In the days following 9/11, various messages released by government officials, health care professionals, scientists, and the media ran the gamut from reports of extremely unsafe levels of outdoor air pollutants to the EPA's statement on September 18, 2001, that "the air was safe to breathe." Public concerns remained, however, because families and workers in the World Trade Center area could see and smell fumes from ongoing fires. At a time when there was immense fear and sorrow, because the disaster was of unprecedented scale for New York City, the disparity between what residents and workers were seeing downtown and what they were hearing on the news led to a great deal of confusion.

In the immediate aftermath of 9/11 families were faced with major decisions regarding return to work and to their homes and their children's return to school. Messages that simply conveyed the facts and were laced with technical jargon without providing context often were alarming to the public.

Consider the following statement: "EPA data indicate there were large increases in hourly levels of PM2.5 at and above the Air Quality Index level of 40 μg/m^3. Some hourly levels were reported as high as 200 μg/m^3." This statement uses technical terms such as "PM2.5" and "Air Quality Index" that are unfamiliar to the public. No interpretation is offered as to the potential health effects of exposure to this level of air pollution, and no historical comparison is cited. It should not be surprising that a fearful audience might conclude that the state of the air quality in and around the World Trade Center site was unsafe.

A message explaining the current levels of exposure in comparison with other urban areas or using New York City's own historical levels provided the public with more relevant, accessible, and understandable information needed for decision making. For example, one could amend the message by stating, "Although these 24-hour levels are higher than desirable, they are similar to background levels of air pollution seen previously in New York City." Placing the information in context creates a message that the audience can comprehend more readily.

PEHSU staff participated in numerous community forums in which potential health risks were discussed and recommendations were offered. These forums provided opportunities for the public to express its concerns and for risk communicators to listen and express empathy. Also, the PEHSU staff at the forums included pediatricians with expertise in environmental threats to children's health. These factors enhanced the public's level of trust and confidence in the information presented. At the forums, PEHSU staff shared its review of environmental testing results from both governmental agencies and private firms and then looked to historical environmental testing results for the same areas. Data before 9/11 revealed historical outdoor levels of 18.4 μg/m^3 for PM2.5 (year 2000 average) and levels of 25 μg/m^3 for PM10 (1998 average). Twenty-four–hour levels for New York City have been reported as high as 89 μg/m^3 for PM2.5 and 121 μg/m^3 for PM10 (1996–2001, pre-9/11). This information indicated that even pre-9/11 levels of particulate matter exceeded the National Ambient Air Quality Standards, most likely reflecting background levels of air pollution in urban areas. Although this information stresses that much work is yet to be done to improve the overall quality of outdoor air, it helped place the World Trade Center exposures in context.

Guidance provided to families explained that long-term health effects were unlikely to result from short-term exposures to particulate matter and noted that acute reversible health effects including asthma exacerbations and eye, ear, nose, and throat irritation were possible. Fact sheets were created specifically outlining World Trade Center–related exposures and potential health risks to children including particulate matter (Box 2), lead, asbestos, polychlorinated biphenyls, volatile organic compounds, and dioxins. These fact sheets were distributed at community forums and through community-based organizations and are also accessible online.

Box 2. Particulate matter fact sheet

What is particulate matter?

Particulate matter is the name or term used to describe a variety of small, microscopic particles in the air. The particles include dust, soot, smoke, and cigarette fumes. Also, byproducts of combustion, or burning, such as sulfur dioxide and nitrogen dioxide, are components of particulate matter. Together, these are often called "outdoor air pollutants" and are a major indicator of overall air quality.

What are the sources of particulate matter?

The major sources of particulate matter include the tailpipes of motor vehicles and the smokestacks of factories; mining, construction and demolition; and fires and natural soil erosion.

What determines a child's level of exposure to particulate matter?

A child's level of exposure to particulate matter depends on the distance of the child's home and school from sources of particulate matter, including major roads, bus stations, and construction sites. In general, cities have higher levels of particulate matter than suburban areas.

What else can affect levels of particulate matter in the air?

Levels of particulate matter are affected by the weather, and levels can change depending on the time of day. High winds help spread particulate matter and can decrease levels of particulate matter in the air. Rain washes particulate matter from the air, lowering air-borne levels of particulate matter. During rush hour, heavy traffic and road congestion result in increased vehicle emissions and higher levels of particulate matter.

How does particulate matter affect the health of children?

Short-term exposure to particulate matter may irritate the eyes, ears, nose, throat, and lungs. Symptoms may include coughing, wheezing, and shortness of breath. These symptoms usually stop when the exposure is removed. Children who have asthma may experience an acute asthma attack or worsening symptoms when exposed to high levels.

Is my child at risk of health effects from exposure to particulate matter after the collapse of the World Trade Center?

Although high levels of particulate matter were present immediately after 9/11, levels steadily decreased and by mid-October were consistent with normal background levels for New York City. Reversible, short-term eye, ear, nose, and throat irritation and asthma were likely during the initial period following the collapse. Long-term health effects are unlikely to result from short-term exposure to particulate matter.

How do we prevent further exposure?
Take steps to minimize exposure to particulate matter:
1. Check outdoor air quality alerts. If outdoor levels are high, keep windows and doors closed to keep out the particles and limit the amount of time children play outdoors.
2. Have the filters in your air conditioning and ventilation systems inspected and changed regularly.
3. Prevent particles from spreading in the air by using a High Efficiency Particulate Air (HEPA) vacuum and damp mops or damp cloths to clean inside your home.

A sample message communicating information about risk incorporating the principles discussed in this article and the risk-communication template is included in Fig. 2. Given what was learned from providing health messages to families in the aftermath of 9/11, the template for communications about risk is a clear and concise way to get a message out to the public. Consultation between medical professionals and experts in a variety of fields including risk communication, environmental health, industrial hygiene, and public health is sometimes necessary in developing these types of messages, particularly in complex situations such as after 9/11.

Discussion: putting principles into practice

Addressing parent and guardian concerns about environmental hazards can pose a challenge to pediatric health care providers. Although they may not view themselves as experts in the field of environmental risk assessment and communication, pediatric providers do have certain inherent qualities that make them ideal for communicating information regarding potential environmental health hazards to families and to the community at large. Pediatric providers are credible sources of information, they are trusted by the families of the children they care for, and they are skilled at discussing delicate information.

Miller and Solomon [1], in an adaptation of the "Seven Cardinal Rules of Risk Communication," describe guidelines for clinicians to consider in their practice when communicating risk. The rules are (1) accept and involve the patient as a legitimate partner; (2) plan carefully and evaluate your efforts; (3) listen to the patient's specific concerns; (4) be honest, frank, and open;

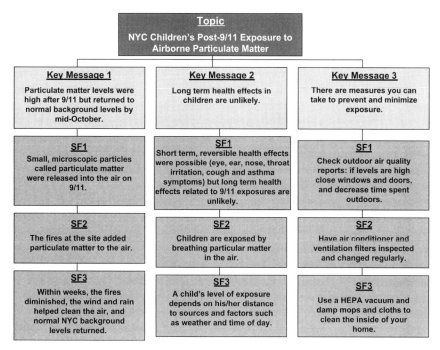

Fig. 2. Sample risk communication message for children's post-9/11 exposure to airborne particulate matter.

(5) coordinate and collaborate with other credible sources; (6) meet the needs of the media; and (7) speak clearly and with compassion [19,20].

Pediatric providers can best advocate for the health of children in the face of environmental disasters, both man-made and natural, by speaking from

---

Box 3. Key lessons learned

1. Focus on factors that can reduce perception of risk, such as providing concrete practical advice that can give the public some level of individual control.
2. In the absence of health-based exposure thresholds, background levels (both present-day and historical) are useful for providing a contextual framework.
3. Use the word "safe" cautiously. Provide specific details: safe for whom, from what, at what time periods, and for how long.
4. Choose risk communicators who carry a high level of public trust such as physicians. Information from independent, academic sources often is viewed as unbiased and reliable.
5. In a time of high concern it is important to craft clear and concise messages, using lay terminology.

their strength as trusted experts on children's health, obtaining the necessary information from experts in allied fields, and developing a clear message that keeps in mind the basic principles of risk communication (Box 3).

Acknowledgments

The authors gratefully acknowledge the invaluable assistance of Damiris Perez, MPA, in the preparation of this article.

References

[1] Miller M, Solomon G. Environmental risk communication for the clinician. Pediatrics 2003; 112:211–7.
[2] Frumkin H. Environmental health from global to local. San Francisco (CA): John Wiley & Sons, Inc.; 2005.
[3] U.S. Environmental Protection Agency. Chemicals-in commerce information system. Chemical update system database. 1998.
[4] Covello VT, Peters RG, Wojtecki JG, et al. Risk communication, the West Nile virus epidemic, and bioterrorism: responding to the communication challenges posed by the intentional or unintentional release of a pathogen in an urban setting. J Urban Health 2001;78:382–91.
[5] National Research Council. Improving risk communication. Washington, DC: National Academy Press; 1989.
[6] Alder P, Kranowitz J. A primer on perceptions of risks, risks communication and building trust. Keystone (CO): The Keystone Center; 2005.
[7] Fischoff B, Slovic P, Lichenstein L, et al. How safe is safe enough? A psychometric study of attitudes towards technological risks and benefits. Policy Sci 1978;9:127–52.
[8] Slovic P. Perception of risk. Science 1987;236:280–5.
[9] Hyer R, Covello V. Effective media communication during public health emergencies: a WHO field guide. Geneva (Switzerland): World Health Organization; 2005.
[10] Peters RG, Covello VT, McCallum DB. The determinants of trust and credibility in environmental risk communication: an empirical study. Risk Anal 1997;17:43–54.
[11] Renn O, Levine D. Credibility and trust in risk communication. Dordrecht (The Netherlands): Kluwer Academic Publishers; 1991. p. 175–281.
[12] Slovic P. Trust, emotion, sex, politics, and science: surveying the risk-assessment battlefield. Risk Anal 1999;19:689–701.
[13] Campbell RG, Babrow AS. The role of empathy in responses to persuasive risk communication: overcoming resistance to HIV prevention messages. Health Commun 2004;16:159–82.
[14] Covello V. Trust & credibility in risk communication. Health & Environment Digest 1992;6: 1–3.
[15] Covello V. Risk communication, trust, and credibility. J Occup Med 1993;35:18–9.
[16] Ong LML, Visser MRM, Lammes FB, et al. Effect of providing cancer patients with the audiotaped initial consultation on satisfaction, recall, and quality of life: a randomized, double-blind study. J Clin Oncol 2000;18(16):3052–60.
[17] Kirschner P. Cognitive load theory: implications of cognitive load theory on the design of learning. Learning and Instruction 2002;12:1–10.
[18] Kahneman D, Tversky A. Prospect theory: an analysis of decision under risk. Econometrica 1979;47:263–91.
[19] Etzel AR, Balk JS, Committee on Environmental Health. Pediatric environmental health. 2nd edition. Elk Grove Village (IL): American Academy of Pediatrics; 2003.
[20] Covello V, Allen F. Seven cardinal rules of risk communication. U.S. Environmental Protection Agency, Office of Policy Analysis; 1992.

ELSEVIER
SAUNDERS

Pediatr Clin N Am
54 (2007) 47–62

PEDIATRIC CLINICS

OF NORTH AMERICA

Environmental Evaluation of a Child with Developmental Disability

Javed Hussain, MD[a,b,c,*],
Alan D. Woolf, MD, MPH[a,b,c,d],
Megan Sandel, MD, MPH[a,c,e],
Michael W. Shannon, MD, MPH[a,b,c,d,f]

[a]*Pediatric Environmental Health Center, Children's Hospital Boston,*
300 Longwood Avenue, Boston, MA 02115, USA
[b]*Harvard Medical School, Boston, MA, USA*
[c]*Pediatric Environmental Health Subspecialty Unit, Children's Hospital Boston,*
300 Longwood Avenue, Boston, MA 02115, USA
[d]*Cambridge Hospital, 1493 Cambridge Street, Cambridge, MA 02139, USA*
[e]*Boston University Medical Center, 1 Boston Medical Center Place, Boston, MA 02118, USA*
[f]*Division of Emergency Medicine, Children's Hospital Boston,*
300 Longwood Avenue, Boston, MA 02115, USA

Environmental pediatrics is an area of pediatric medicine that has been evolving gradually for the past 50 years. Its importance has increased as the industrialized nations have gained good control over major infectious diseases and have been increasingly faced with chronic conditions, such as asthma, cancer, and developmental disabilities. There has been growing recognition that chemicals in the environment are responsible, at least in part, for these striking changes in the patterns of childhood diseases [1]. A child's health is associated closely with the environment in which he or she lives; the child's health can be affected adversely by unfavorable exposure to these chemical agents.

The growth of children's environmental health as a discipline in pediatric medicine has been fueled by the evidence that the fetus and young children are particularly vulnerable to environmental influences. Children have unique patterns of environmental exposure and developmentally determined

This work was supported in part by a grant from the ATSDR Superfund Reconciliation & Reclamation Act, administered through the Association of Occupational and Environmental Clinics Association (AOEC), Washington, DC.

* Corresponding author. Division of General Pediatrics, Children's Hospital Boston, 300 Longwood Avenue, Boston, MA 02115.

E-mail address: javed.hussain@childrens.harvard.edu (J. Hussain).

susceptibilities that increase their risk of disease following contact with environmental agents [2]. These age groups are more sensitive because of factors including (1) their low body weight, (2) the likelihood that they will come into contact with environmental toxins because they are closer to the floor and ground where many toxins are more concentrated, (3) their increased respiratory rates, and (4) their tendency to bring whatever they have in their hands into their mouths [3]. Children also have more prospective years of life left than adults; thus they have a longer time in which to develop the complications of toxin-related injury suffered in pregnancy, infancy, or childhood.

The developing human central nervous system is the target organ most vulnerable to environmental toxins [4], and a number of agents have been shown to have neurotoxic effects either in human or experimental studies. Critical windows of vulnerability to the effects of these agents occur pre- and postnatally. The nervous system is relatively unique in that different areas are responsible for different functional domains (eg, motor control, sensory function, intelligence, and executive function), and these areas develop at different times. In addition, the many cell types in the brain have different windows of vulnerability with varying sensitivities to environmental agents [5]. Neurulation begins early in embryogenesis with formation of the neural plate at 2 weeks of gestation [6]. The first neurons, formed during the middle of the first trimester of pregnancy, proliferate and differentiate while migrating to patterned final destinations in the nervous system. Programmed cell death (apoptosis), neurotrophic factors, and, at a molecular level, signal transduction are other processes that modulate this cascading process of neuronal matrix formation [6]. Glial cells also proliferate during the second trimester of fetal life, coating the neurons with protective myelin, which allows more efficient signal transmission. Myelination continues through adolescence, although 80% of the adult brain's weight is achieved by 6 years of age [7]. Synaptogenesis and neurotransmitter production continues to build the connectivity of the neuronal architecture through the first 2 years of life. Any of these stages and processes of brain development are subject to disruption by the injurious effects (either direct toxicity or downstream consequences) of exogenous toxicants, such as radiation, noise, ethanol, solvents, pesticides, polychlorinated biphenyls (PCBs) and dioxin, lead, methyl mercury, and other pollutants. At the same time, neuroplasticity may allow compensatory recovery of some functions after neurologic injury throughout childhood and adolescence.

The scope of child exposure to environmental agents is enormous. More than 80,000 chemicals are permitted in the United States; an increasing number are used in everyday consumer products [8]. Three to 4 million children and adolescents in the United States live within 1 mile of a federally designated Superfund site and are at risk of exposure to chemical toxicants released from these sites into air, groundwater, surface water, and soil; all of these factors can affect surrounding (or even distant) communities [9].

Considerable evidence has accumulated during the last 2 decades indicating that low-level exposure to environmental toxicants and pollutants may be associated with adverse effects including preterm birth, reduced birth weight, lowered intelligence, poor school performance, and increased rates of behavioral problems.

Epidemiology

Approximately 17% of individuals in the United States 18 years and younger have a developmental disability, and for most children the cause of the condition is unknown [10]. Developmental disabilities are characterized by physical, cognitive, psychologic, sensory, adaptive, and/ or communication impairments manifested during early child development. Developmental disabilities exert a great social and financial impact. For example, new data indicate that even low levels of lead exposure produce subtle deficits in IQ, which can have significant societal impact when large numbers of children are affected. A 1 μg/dL decrease in blood lead concentration in children in the United States who have blood lead concentrations between 10 and 20 μg/dL would translate into a savings of $5 billion to $7.5 billion a year in increased earning power alone [11].

Three major developmental disabilities, autism, cerebral palsy (CP), and severe mental retardation, affect substantial numbers of children in United States. Very little is known about the etiology of these conditions. The prevalence of childhood conditions such as learning disabilities, attention deficit hyperactivity disorder (ADHD), and autistic spectrum disorder (ASD) has risen remarkably during the past 30 years. CDC estimates based on two national health surveys, conducted in 2003–2004, that about 5.6 per 1000 children aged 4–17 had a parent reported autism disorder [12]. ASD includes five conditions of varying severity ranging from autism to pervasive developmental disorder. Under the criteria in the *Diagnostic and Statistical Manual of Mental Disorders,* fourth edition, this spectrum of disorders is characterized by restricted communication skills, impairment of reciprocal social interaction, and a restricted/repetitive pattern of interest and/or behavior. CP is a heterogeneous group of nonprogressive clinical syndromes that is characterized by motor and postural dysfunction. In the last 40 years the prevalence of CP has risen to well above 2 per 1000 live births. A large proportion of children who have CP have some degree of cognitive impairment; the prevalence of intellectual deficits varies with the type of CP and increases significantly when epilepsy is present [13]. Mental retardation is another heterogeneous group of conditions defined by significantly below-average intellectual and adaptive functioning and onset before age 18 years [14]. The prevalence of mental retardation in the general population is estimated to be approximately 1%.

Learning disabilities are a heterogeneous group of disorders characterized by the unexpected failure of an individual to acquire, retrieve, and use information competently that results in academic achievement at a level less than expected for the individual's intellectual potential [15]. Learning disabilities are caused by inborn or acquired abnormalities in brain structure and function; they often have a multifactorial etiology. Learning disabilities are not a single disorder. The category includes disabilities in any of seven areas related to reading, language, and mathematics. These separate types of learning disabilities frequently co-occur with one another and with social deficits and emotional and behavioral problems, including ADHD. Childhood placement in learning disability programs in the United States has tripled during the last few decades, rising to 6%. In 1997 and 1998 the National Health Interview Survey reported a diagnosis of learning disability in 4% of children between the ages of 6 and 11 years [16].

ADHD is a condition that can affect cognitive, academic, behavioral, emotional, and social functioning. It commonly manifests in early childhood with symptoms of inattention, hyperactivity, and impulsivity. The prevalence of ADHD in the United States is estimated to range from 4% to 6% in children between the ages of 4 and 17 years [17]. Its prevalence, however, may be as high as 8% to 10% in school-aged children; ADHD can persist into adulthood in more then 70% of afflicted children [18]. Its etiology is unknown.

Putative etiologies

The vulnerability of the human central nervous system to environmental chemicals has been well established, but the contribution these exposures may make to problems such as ADHD, conduct problems, mental retardation, learning disabilities, or ASD remains uncertain. The environmental neurotoxicants that have been shown to produce developmental neurotoxicity in rigorous, reproducible investigations include PCBs, dioxins, pesticides, ionizing radiation, environmental tobacco smoke, and in utero exposure to alcohol, tobacco, marijuana, and cocaine. Exposure to these environmental agents can result in a spectrum of adverse outcomes from severe mental retardation and learning disabilities to more subtle changes in function depending on the timing and dose of the chemical agent [5].

Lead

Childhood exposure to high doses of lead can result in encephalopathy and convulsions. Lower-dose lead exposures have been associated with impairment in intellectual function, speech, language, behavior, and attention [5].

Methyl mercury

High-dose prenatal exposure to methyl mercury can produce mental retardation, CP, and visual and auditory deficits in children of exposed mothers. At lower levels of exposure, the observed effects may be subtler.

There is little evidence that mercury exposure is responsible for the rising prevalence of ASD in children. Although openly acknowledging the limitations of current scientific knowledge, pediatricians should remain skeptical of simple explanations offered as a single root cause of children's complex developmental disabilities. The National Academy of Sciences, for example, upon completion of an exhaustive review of the extant scientific literature, could find no association between exposure to thimerosal and autism [19]. Hviid and colleagues [20] studied two groups of children born in Denmark between 1990 and 1996. One group was vaccinated with thimerosal-containing vaccine; the other group received thimerosal-free vaccine. The investigators found no causal relationship between childhood vaccination, use of thimerosal-containing vaccine, and development of an ASD. Many other studies failed to demonstrate a link between thimerosal-containing vaccines and ASD [21,22].

Polychlorinated biphenyls

PCBs are industrial chemicals that were used widely in the manufacture of transformers and other electrical devices. After approximately 50 years use, they were banned in 1977 [23]. Some PCB-containing products are still in use, however, and others have been disposed of in landfills and industrial disposal sites. PCBs also are found in river sludge as a result of past water discharges during manufacture and disposal. Because of their extremely slow biodegradation, these products remain ubiquitous in the environment, the food chain, and human fatty tissue. High-level in utero exposures to PCB can cause developmental deficits accompanied by growth retardation [24]. The threshold for this toxicity is unclear, however [25].

Pesticides, alcohol, and metals

Pesticides are an extremely heterogeneous group of substances. Most are synthetic chemicals manufactured specifically for their toxic properties to the target species. Several epidemiologic studies in the United States have suggested health concerns arising from the chronic exposure of young children to pesticides in the domestic environment [26]. For example, dichloro diphenyl trichloroethane (DDT) is an organochlorine pesticide that, like PCB, was banned years ago. DDT is a proven "neuroendocrine disrupter" as well as a "functional teratogen" that can lead to harmful effects on brain development and the timing of puberty [27,28].

Alcohol is a well-established teratogen. Heavy exposure to alcohol in utero is associated with fetal alcohol syndrome. Mental retardation is one of the main symptoms of fetal alcohol syndrome [29]. Teratogenic, cognitive, or behavior effects associated with prenatal exposure to other substances (eg, marijuana, tobacco, cocaine, or opiates) have been less clearly established. With in utero exposure, several of these agents produce significant intrauterine growth retardation. Impaired fetal growth, particularly when head growth is affected, may affect cognition indirectly [30].

Metals like aluminum are neurotoxicants to both animals and humans. Manganese has been associated with neurotoxicity in adults and children [31].

Evaluation of the child who has developmental delay from suspected environmental exposure

Children who have developmental disabilities that are suspected to result from exposure to an environmental agent should undergo a complete evaluation that includes a detailed history, a physical examination, and a diagnostic work-up (Boxes 1 and 2).

Environmental history

An accurate history obtained from one or more members of the family is a vital part of the environmental evaluation. In the assessment of developmental disability caused by a possible environmental neurotoxicant, a detailed and accurate review of the presenting illness is very important. The environmental history can be broadly subdivided into nine different sections (see Box 1).

Prenatal history

A chronic illness in the mother, such as diabetes, can adversely affect the nervous system of the child [32]. Antiepileptic drugs also may affect the fetus. For example, valproic acid and hydantoin may disrupt neural tube development and can cause congenital malformation and mental retardation. A significant exposure to lead in the mother can lead to excess exposure to the fetus that may result in mental retardation and developmental delay in the infant [33]. It also is important to inquire about the type and amount of fish consumption by the mother during pregnancy. Evidence from an outbreak of methyl mercury poisoning in Iraq suggested that adverse effects of prenatal exposure on child development begin to appear at or above 10 ppm measured in maternal hair [34]. Exposure of the fetus to ionizing radiation during early pregnancy results in an increased risk for microcephaly and other adverse outcomes [35]. Exposure to arsenic during pregnancy may result in spontaneous abortion or low birth weight [36]. Alcohol consumption during pregnancy increases the risk of mental retardation as part of a recognizable pattern of congenital abnormalities known as fetal alcohol syndrome.

Birth history

The length of the pregnancy and any complications during labor or delivery should be explored. Children born prematurely or who have intrauterine growth retardation have a higher incidence of developmental disabilities such as mental retardation, learning disabilities, and CP [37]. Birth weight,

---

Box 1. General history of a child with developmental disability

Prenatal history: chronic medical conditions, medications, tobacco use, alcohol or substance use, exposure to heavy metals

Birth history: gestational age, birth weight, Apgar score, perinatal problems, postpartum length of hospital stay

Early developmental milestones: age of sitting up without support, walking unassisted, first spoken word, combining words

Neurodevelopment: previous neurodevelopmental evaluations in chronologic orders

Current level of developmental function: Language (expressive and receptive), cognition, motor function (gross and fine), activity level, behavior

Past medical history: hospitalizations, sick visits to primary care physician or emergency department, injuries or infections, surgeries, immunizations, list of all practitioners other than primary care physician involved in care, list of all previous laboratory evaluations, list of all previous therapies, including chelation, megavitamins, dietary supplements

Diet: history of use of unusual or unconventional diet, general description of current diet

Medication and allergies: allergies, past and present medications, current dietary supplements

Potential environmental exposure: at home any pesticide use, recent renovation, water source, type of heating, types of any hobbies practiced within the home, any environmental assessment, carbon monoxide detector; any industries in the vicinity, and nature of their operation; list of all previous lead tests, presence of mercury on premises, any potential environmental exposures in the neighborhood.

Apgar score, perinatal problems, and the postnatal course may be important pieces of data in ruling in or ruling out potential causes of problems in the young child.

Early developmental history

Developmental milestones should be reviewed and recorded. The milestones of greatest importance include the age at which the child sat without support, walked unassisted, spoke his/her first words, and began to combine words. The history of language and speech acquisition should be reviewed, along with an inventory of current developmental function. Such a history should include estimates of current expressive and receptive language skills

Box 2. Family history

Maternal history
Age at patient's birth, parity, any fetal loss
Diet and infections or hospitalizations during pregnancy
Cigarette, alcohol, or substance abuse during pregnancy
Dietary supplements, including alternative remedies and
    medications, during pregnancy
Dental work
Need for anti-D immunoglobulins
Occupation: current and during pregnancy
Educational attainment
History of learning difficulties
Relatives who have neurodevelopmental disorders

Paternal history
Age at patient's birth
Prior children and their current health
Use of medications or dietary supplements before pregnancy
Tobacco, alcohol, or substance use before pregnancy
Educational attainment
Occupational history
History of learning difficulties
Relatives who have neurodevelopmental disorders

Sibling history
Name and ages of all siblings
Current level of developmental function of all siblings

as well as accurate details of cognitive abilities and gross and fine motor function. Certain details of the child's behavior (eg, a history of pica) suggest the potential exposure to an environmental toxicant.

Many children who later present with delayed development have had feeding problems, excessive colic, frequent formula changes, and abnormal sleeping patterns; these pieces of data might also be useful [38].

Neurodevelopmental assessment history

A list of all prior neurobehavioral evaluations should be obtained in chronologic order. The outcome of the evaluation and intervention offered should be documented.

Past medical history

A careful review of the past medial history should focus on major childhood illnesses, surgery, injuries, and immunizations. Recurrent injuries suggest hyperactivity, impaired coordination, or poor impulse control. A list of all the practitioners involved in the care of the child, including consultation with any alternative providers (eg, naturopaths, acupuncturists, or Ayurvedic practitioners), should be recorded. All laboratory evaluations that have been performed should be noted. Any previous therapies used to treat the child's condition, including chelation, megavitamins, and dietary supplements, should be documented.

Diet and medication

The clinician must determine what medications the child is taking or has taken as well as any unusual dietary supplements or restricted diet plans that the child follows.

Potential environmental exposures

A detailed history of the home environment, day care, and any other residence where the child spends time is important. The age of the house, its composition, and any recent renovations may reveal toxic hazards. Very young children and children who have developmental disabilities have a risk of becoming exposed to lead paint and dust, producing significant lead exposure. The family's water source should be ascertained. Well water could be a source of lead, aluminum, mercury, manganese, PCB, or other contaminants. The presence of an industry, gasoline station, or dry cleaner in close proximity to the child's home increases the potential for exposure to leaked materials or industrial waste in ground and surface water and also can affect ambient air quality. Broken thermostats or thermometers or the use of mercury for ritual purposes in the household could be a source of contamination. Any other potential environmental exposures, including proximity to a nearby landfill, should be investigated. Inquiry into the type of home heating could reveal evidence of exposure to carbon monoxide or nitrogen oxides. A history of using cleansers, pesticides, or other chemicals should lead to concern about exposure to solvents or volatile organic compounds.

Family history

A detailed family history (see Box 2) should include the mother's age at the time of delivery, parity, and diet. A maternal history of cigarette smoking or alcohol and substance abuse during pregnancy is also key information. Important elements of the paternal history should include preconception use of medications, substances of abuse, or occupational hazards. Document the ages and developmental function of all siblings.

Physical assessment

The child's height, weight, and head circumference should be measured. The presence of any dysmorphic features in the child's general appearance should be noted. Careful observation should be made of the child's behaviors (activity, speech, and interactions with other family members). The appearance of the skull can suggest the presence of microcephaly or macro-cephaly. Flattening of the occiput can be seen in developmentally delayed children. The location of the hair whorl and the appearance of palmar creases always should be noted. Abnormalities of whorl pattern can indicate the presence of a cerebral malformation. The diagnostician also should in-vestigate the child's oral hygiene and condition of the teeth. Prolonged, high levels of lead exposure may result in the development of lead lines at the junction of gums and teeth. Attention should be paid to skin for lesions such as café-au-lait spots, angiomas, or areas of hypopigmentation, which could be clues to neurologic disorders. Examination of the chest, heart, and abdomen, and the musculoskeletal and nervous systems always should be part of the general physical examination.

Environmental data and their interpretation

Environmental data can be separated into two main sections: biologic (testing of the patient) and environmental. It is important to acknowledge that more advanced testing is often in the research and not the clinical realm. Often testing in the environment is used to determine the source of the exposure but does not necessarily prove that a child was exposed to toxins discovered in the environment.

Use and interpretation of laboratory data

As all medical students are taught, data gathered from the history is the most important element in assessing possible environmental exposures. The physician should avoid the temptation of a shot-gun approach to testing without substantial suspicion raised by the thorough history and physical examination. With the limited amount of biologic testing that can be done in the clinical setting of environmental health, it is important to under-stand and explain accurately what results can and cannot confirm. Often, testing can show only recent exposure and cannot easily show long-term exposure. Also, exposure often may have occurred in the prenatal period, which would require testing at that time, not at a later date. For example, testing for acute or recent exposure to pesticides does not rule out a long-term exposure or a history of an acute exposure in the past.

Sometimes it becomes essential to run series of tests such as blood lead level to monitor suspected exposure or clearance of the chemical from the body or to assess the effect of chelation therapy. Most environmental toxicants, how-ever, do not have a simple blood test, and confirming the suspected exposure relies on testing of the ambient environment. Testing for mercury, pesticides, and PCBs should be performed in a specialized setting.

Finally, laboratory data from commercial laboratories other than those within a certified hospital or public health department should be reviewed carefully, because many laboratories use unconventional testing methods and interpretations. Often the data they provide is misleading and inaccurate. Parents should be discouraged from seeking out unproven diagnostic measures, such as extensive analyses of hair for metals and trace elements. Recent studies have shown that sample collection and the technical aspects of analysis may lead to wide variations in test results, without good evidence of accuracy or reliability [39,40]. The minerals and metals assayed may not have been studied in populations of children so as to create normal reference ranges [39,41]. Biologic variability of the deposition of minerals and metals in hair must be studied further with respect to kinetics, ethnic and racial variations, and age-related fluctuations [41]. The results of such assays often have no known correlation with clinical diagnoses.

Treatment, counseling, and prevention

Chelation therapy

In children who have developmental delays that are suspected to result from exposure to an environmental toxicant, discussions about chelation therapy often ensue. Defined as the administration of an agent that will enhance the elimination of a stored toxin, chelation is a treatment most commonly used for exposure to lead, arsenic, iron, and, occasionally, mercury. There are several chelating agents available, administered orally or parenterally.

Although chelation has long been shown to have value in select children who have lead or iron intoxication, its role in the treatment of other intoxications or disorders is unproven. For example, chelation therapy to eliminate mercury in children who have autism has become an increasingly popular although discredited intervention. Its use is based on the belief that mercury exposure, from mercury-containing products ranging from seafood to dental amalgam to thimerosal, can produce a clinical picture identical to the ASD. Currently there is a community of practitioners and parents of children who have ASD who firmly believe that chelation therapy can produce significant developmental benefits. The most common chelation agents being used in children who have ASD are parenteral calcium disodium ethylenediaminetetraacetic acid (CaNa2EDTA), and the oral medication, succimer. Although the Food and Drug Administration has approved succimer for oral administration only, it often is reformulated (compounded) by practitioners and administered rectally or transdermally, practices that are unsafe and should be discouraged.

According to generally accepted principles indicating chelation therapy, the administration of chelants to most children who have ASD is inappropriate. Chelation therapy should follow the principles outlined in Box 3. The American Academy of Pediatrics, in a recent policy statement addressing the evaluation and management of children who have ASD, recommended against the routine chelation of such children [42].

Box 3. Principles of chelation

1. Laboratory and clinical evidence that the patient has a metal intoxication. In case of laboratory evidence, the measurement must be performed using conventional assays and must be quantitative, yielding a numeric value that will be monitored through the course of chelation.
2. The goals of chelation are clear and quantitative. For example, when chelation therapy is undertaken for lead intoxication, there is an established goal at the outset for the blood lead level desired.
3. The chelator, in the form administered, is proven to chelate the toxicant in question. Chelating agents differ greatly in their properties and in their ability to bind metals.
4. The benefits of chelation therapy will exceed any risks. All chelating agents, like all drugs, have adverse effects associated with their use. The adverse effects include allergic reaction, hepatotoxicity, renal injury, and depletion of essential nutrients.

Complementary and alternative medicine therapies

Families of children who have developmental delays or autism often are faced with an indeterminate diagnosis, caused by an unknown etiology and carrying with it an uncertain future. They understandably seek a variety of opinions and, sometimes, try novel therapies to improve their child's health and enhance his or her developmental progress. There is no end of advice offered by well-meaning family, friends, advocacy groups, and in popular magazines or via the Internet. Families are influenced easily by inspiring testimonials, plausible theories of causation, and fantastic claims of success.

Previous studies have shown that parents of children who have a chronic disease use complementary and alternative medicine (CAM) therapies more frequently than do parents of children who have no such health problems. Rather than being disenchanted or antagonistic to allopathic medicine, many parents integrate conventional medical management options with CAM therapies in a continuing quest for a better functional outcome for their child [43]. Some CAM therapies, such as behavioral modification, biofeedback, sensory integration techniques, music, therapeutic massage, spirituality, and mind-body techniques, have varying degrees of scientific evidence of their value but may indeed be salutary adjunctive measures for patients who have developmental delays, autism, or mental retardation.

Frustration with the perceived ineffectiveness of conventional medical, psychologic, and/or educational management options may drive some parents to consider CAM therapies for their children. Such therapies also may be more aligned with parents' own sociocultural and ethnic backgrounds or more consistent with their personal lifestyle choices and philosophy about health care. Many are attracted to the sense of control these therapies give them over their child's condition; they may feel more supported and more effective as advocates for their child. They may perceive herbs, homeopathic or ethnic remedies, special diets, and dietary supplements to be more natural (and therefore safe) and associated with fewer side effects than prescribed or over-the-counter medications [44]. There are, however, case reports of severe toxicity resulting from the use of herbal treatments in children who have developmental delays. For example, an aphasic boy who had severe mental retardation, CP, and a seizure disorder was rendered comatose by an Asian patent remedy containing significant amounts of both bromides and barbiturates [45].

Complementary and alternative medicine and family counseling

Pediatric health care providers may avoid discussing parents' use of the use of CAM therapies for their children because they are not confident about their own knowledge of such therapies [46]. They also may be perceived by parents as having a closed mind or as being openly hostile to the choice of CAM for children. Parents may feel that the pediatrician would not understand, support, or approve their pursuit of such options as an integral part of their child's care.

A recent review of the safety and effectiveness of herbs and dietary supplements provided guidance on how to counsel families regarding the use of CAM for their children [47]. Eisenberg [43] has proposed that, when considering questions of the safety and effectiveness of a particular CAM therapy, health professionals use the guide: "Would I recommend this therapy for my family member?" There are several reliable sources of information about CAM for practitioners. The first is the National Center for Complementary and Alternative Medicine (NCCAM) of the National Institutes of Health (http://nccam.nih.gov/health/). From the NCCAM website, one can link to the Herbs and Supplements database of MEDLINEplus, which is compiled by the National Library of Medicine. The National Institutes of Health also has an Office of Dietary Supplements (http://dietary-supplements.info.nih.gov/). From that page one can link to several additional databases.

Counseling parents after an environmental evaluation

Families of children who have developmental disorders often have preconceived opinions about its cause and about what measures will improve their child's condition. On the Internet they may have encountered troubling information about the association of autism with toxins such as mercury. They previously may have consulted alternative practitioners who, after hair testing or other dubious assessments, have convinced them that a particular toxin accounts for their child's condition and must be rectified by scientifically unproven interventions (eg, dietary modifications, chelants, immunotherapy, herbs, dietary supplements, laxatives, vitamins).

They may seek validation of their approach to their child's care by the pediatric health care provider and value that judgment and approval. Alternatively they may have less therapeutic motivations, such as justifying insurance claims or legal actions. Some families are motivated by the desire to confirm their perception of the inadequacies of allopathic medicine. There may well be a need to vent frustration, stress, and anger at the family's current situation of uncertainty.

The pediatrician's role in such encounters should be one of open-mindedness, understanding, and support, with sensitivity to a family's particular set of health beliefs and practices that may reflect cultural and ethnic differences. The health care provider, however, must take care to strike a balance between well-intended listening, counseling, and support versus an appearance of acquiescence to management plans that may be harmful to the child. Collusion with the family in the pursuit of remedies that have no known scientific basis offers at best only added expense, placebo-related outcomes, and false hopes. At worst such practices may fundamentally betray the family's trust, subject the child to unnecessary risks, and confound the pursuit of the child's best medical interests.

Summary

This article reviews the prevalence and reputed environmental etiologies of developmental disabilities among children in the United States. There has been growing recognition that chemicals in the environment may be contributing at least in part to these disabilities. Media attention to conditions such as autism may contribute to the anxiety in parents and caregivers who are taking care of the children who have these disabilities. Practitioners treating children who have disabilities can help parents and caregivers by investigating plausible environmental etiologies.

References

[1] Landrigan PJ. Children's environmental health. Lessons from the past and prospects for the future. Pediatr Clin North Am 2001;48:1319–30.
[2] Landrigan PJ. Children as a vulnerable population. Int J Occup Med Environ Health 2004; 17:175–7.
[3] Matsuzaki K. The holding of "International Symposium on Children's Environmental Health". Nippon Eiseigaku Zasshi 2005;60:70–6.
[4] Dietrich KN, Eskenazi B, Schantz S, et al. Principles and practices of neurodevelopmental assessment in children: lessons learned from the centers for children's environmental health and disease prevention research. Environ Health Perspect 2005;113:1437–46.
[5] Mendola P, Selevan SG, Gutter S, et al. Environmental factors associated with a spectrum of neurodevelopmental deficits. Ment Retard Dev Disabil Res Rev 2002;8:188–97.

[6] Rice D, Barone S Jr. Critical periods of vulnerability for the developing nervous system: evidence from humans and animal models. Environ Health Perspect 2000; 108(Suppl 3):511–33.

[7] Grandjean P, White R. Neurodevelopmental disorders. In: Children's health and environment: a review of evidence. Environmental Issue Report No. 29. Copenhagen (Denmark): WHO/European Environment Agency; 2002.

[8] Schaefer M. Children and toxic substances: confronting a major public health challenge. Environ Health Perspect 1994;102(Suppl 2):155–6.

[9] Landrigan PJ, Suk WA, Amler RW. Chemical wastes, children's health, and the Superfund Basic Research Program. Environ Health Perspect 1999;107:423–7.

[10] Rice C, Schendel D, Cunniff C, et al. Public health monitoring of developmental disabilities with a focus on the autism spectrum disorders. Am J Med Genet C Semin Med Genet 2004; 125:22–7.

[11] Rice DC. Issues in developmental neurotoxicology: interpretation and implications of the data. Can J Public Health 1998;89(Suppl 1):S31–40.

[12] Fact Sheet. CDC Autism Research. May 4, 2006. Available at: http://www.cdc.gov/od/oc/media/transcripts/AutismResearchFactSheet.pdf.

[13] Odding E, Roebroeck ME, Stam HJ. The epidemiology of cerebral palsy: incidence, impairments and risk factors. Disabil Rehabil 2006;28:183–91.

[14] Szymanski L, King BH. Practice parameters for the assessment and treatment of children, adolescents, and adults with mental retardation and comorbid mental disorders. American Academy of Child and Adolescent Psychiatry Working Group on Quality Issues. J Am Acad Child Adolesc Psychiatry 1999;38:5S.

[15] Adelman HS. LD: the next 25 years. J Learn Disabil 1992;25:17S–31S.

[16] Pastor PN, Reuben CA. Attention deficit disorder and learning disability: United States, 1997–98. Vital Health Stat 10 2002 May;(206):1–12.

[17] Cuffe SP, Moore CG, McKeown RE. Prevalence and correlates of ADHD symptoms in the National Health Interview Survey. J Atten Disord 2005;9:392–401.

[18] Kessler RC, Adler L, Barkley R, et al. The prevalence and correlates of adult ADHD in the United States: results from the National Comorbidity Survey Replication. Am J Psychiatry 2006;163(4):716–23.

[19] Immunization Safety Review Committee (ISRC). Immunization safety review: vaccines & autism. Washington, DC: National Academy of Science; 2004.

[20] Hviid A, Stellfeld M, Wohlfahrt J, et al. Association between thimerosal containing vaccine and autism. JAMA 2003;290(13):1763–6.

[21] Parker S, Todd J, Schwartz B, et al. Thimerosal-containing vaccines and autistic spectrum disorder: a critical review of published original data. Pediatrics 2005;115(1):200. erratum for Pediatrics 2004;114(3):793–804.

[22] McMahon WM. Review: vaccines containing thimerosal are not associated with autistic spectrum disorders in children. Evid Based Ment Health 2005;8(1):23.

[23] Agency for Toxic Substances and Disease Registry. Polychorinated bipheynls (PCB) toxicity. In: Case studies in environmental medicine, course SS3067, page 7. Revised September 2000.

[24] Hertz-Picciotto I, Charles MJ, James RA, et al. In utero polychlorinated biphenyl exposures in relation to fetal and early childhood growth. Epidemiology 2005;16:648–56.

[25] Rice DC. Neurotoxicity of lead, methylmercury, and PCBs in relation to the Great Lakes. Environ Health Perspect 1995;103(Suppl 9):71–87.

[26] Grey CN, Nieuwenhuijsen MJ, Golding J. The use and disposal of household pesticides. Environ Res 2005;97:109–15.

[27] Dorner G, Plagemann A. DDT in human milk and mental capacities in children at school age: an additional view on PISA 2000. Neuro Endocrinol Lett 2002;23:427–31.

[28] Parent AS, Rasier G, Gerard A, et al. Early onset of puberty: tracking genetic and environmental factors. Horm Res 2005;64(Suppl 2):41–7.

[29] Chiriboga CA. Fetal alcohol and drug effects. Neurologist 2003;9:267–79.
[30] Chiriboga CA, Bateman DA, Hauser WA, et al. Neurologic findings in neonates with intra-uterine cocaine exposure. Pediatr Neurol 1993;9(2):115–9.
[31] Fell JM, Reynolds AP, Meadows N, et al. Manganese toxicity in children receiving long-term parenteral nutrition. Lancet 1996;347:1218–21.
[32] Sells CJ, Robinson NM, Brown Z, et al. Long-term developmental follow-up of infants of diabetic mothers. J Pediatr 1994;125:S9–17.
[33] Goma A, Hu H, Bellinger D, et al. Maternal bone lead as an independent risk factor for fetal neurotoxicity: a prospective study. Pediatrics 2002;110:110–8.
[34] Davidson PW, Myers GJ, Weiss B, et al. Prenatal methyl mercury exposure from fish consumption and child development: a review of evidence and perspectives from the Seychelles Child Development Study. Neurotoxicology 2006;27(6):1106–9.
[35] Streffer C. Bystander effects, adaptive response and genomic instability induced by prenatal irradiation. Mutat Res 2004;568:79–87.
[36] Domingo JL. Prevention by chelating agents of metal-induced developmental toxicity. Reprod Toxicol 1995;9:105–13.
[37] Lorenz JM. The outcome of extreme prematurity. Semin Perinatol 2001;25:348–59.
[38] Menkes JH, Moser FG. Neurological examination of the child and infant. In: Menkes Sarnet, Maria, editors. Text book of child neurology. 7th edition. Lippincott Williams & Wilkins; 2006. p. 1–2.
[39] Seidel S, Kreutzer R, Smith D, et al. Assessment of commercial laboratories performing hair mineral analysis. JAMA 2001;285:67–72.
[40] Steindel SJ, Howanitz PJ. The uncertainty of hair analysis for trace metals. JAMA 2001;285:83–5.
[41] Harkins DK, Susten AS. Hair analysis: exploring the state of the science. Environ Health Perspect 2003;111:576–8.
[42] American Academy of Pediatrics Committee on Children With Disabilities. Technical Report. The pediatrician's role in the diagnosis and management of autistic spectrum disorder in children. Pediatrics 2001;107.
[43] Eisenberg DM. Advising patients who seek alternative medical therapies. Ann Intern Med 1997;127:61–9.
[44] Astin JA. Why patients use alternative medicine: results of a national study. JAMA 1998;279(19):1548–53.
[45] Boyer EW, Kearney S, Shannon MW, et al. Poisoning from a dietary supplement administered during hospitalization. Pediatrics 2002;109(3):E49.
[46] Woolf AD, Gardiner P, Whelan J, et al. Views of pediatric health care providers on the use of herbs and dietary supplements in children. Clin Pediatr (Phila) 2005;44:579–87.
[47] Woolf AD. Herbal remedies and children: do they work? Are they harmful? Pediatrics 2003;112:240–6.

ELSEVIER
SAUNDERS

Pediatr Clin N Am
54 (2007) 63–80

PEDIATRIC CLINICS
OF NORTH AMERICA

Health Effects of Common Home, Lawn, and Garden Pesticides

Catherine J. Karr, MD, PhD, MS[a,b,c,*],
Gina M. Solomon, MD, MPH[d,e],
Alice C. Brock-Utne, MD[f]

[a]Department of Pediatrics, University of Washington, Seattle, WA, USA
[b]Department of Environmental & Occupational Health Sciences,
University of Washington, Seattle, WA, USA
[c]Pediatric Environmental Health Specialty Unit, University of Washington, Seattle, WA, USA
[d]Pediatric Environmental Health Specialty Unit,
University of California at San Francisco, San Francisco, CA, USA
[e]Natural Resources Defense Council, San Francisco, CA, USA
[f]University of California at San Francisco, San Francisco, CA, USA

Pesticides are a source of concern and confusion for both parents and health care providers. This confusion reflects the diversity of products available and their widespread use where children live, go to school, play, and in the food supply coupled with evolving evidence of potential harm from cumulative exposure. The National Home and Garden Pesticide Use Survey conducted by the US Environmental Protection Agency (EPA) found that 82% of households in the United States use pesticides, with an average of three to four different pesticide products used per home [1]. A landmark review in 1993 by the National Academy of Sciences concluded that children may be especially vulnerable to adverse health effects from pesticides [2]. In the last decade studies have demonstrated that the biologic mechanisms underlying this increased susceptibility include both behavioral and developmental factors that can increase the dose and toxicity children experience as compared with adults [3]. Recent studies in pediatric populations have begun to address multiple routes of exposure, exposure to multiple pesticides, and the influence of gene–environment interactions [4–6]. Population-based surveys by the Centers for Disease Control and Prevention have reported

* Corresponding author. University of Washington, Occupational & Environmental Medicine Program, Box 359739, 325 9th Avenue, Seattle, WA 98104.
E-mail address: ckarr@u.washington.edu (C.J. Karr).

0031-3955/07/$ - see front matter © 2007 Elsevier Inc. All rights reserved.
doi:10.1016/j.pcl.2006.11.005
pediatric.theclinics.com

the pervasive presence of a variety of pesticides in the blood and urine of children in the U.S. The third National Report on Human Exposure to Environmental Chemicals, released in July 2005, included testing of 44 pesticide metabolites in a sample representative of the civilian, noninstitutionalized U.S. population over age six years. Of these chemicals, 29 were detectable in most people sampled, with organophosphate and organochlorine insecticides reported to be most prevalent in the population [7].

The pediatric health burden of pesticide exposure includes both acute and chronic health impacts. Acute symptoms range from mild and subtle to severe (eg, nausea, headaches, skin rashes, eye irritation, seizures, coma, and death). Chronic conditions associated with pesticides in epidemiologic studies of children include birth defects, cancer, asthma, and neurodevelopmental/neurobehavioral effects.

Case study

On the day her house was sprayed, a full-term, previously healthy 4-month-old girl became irritable and congested in her upper airway with a thick, whitish nasal discharge. Over the next several days these symptoms persisted; she began to refuse food, she developed a fever and more frequent bowel movements, and her sleep decreased. On day 6 she was brought to the emergency department, received intravenous fluids for hypernatremia and dehydration, and was discharged with a diagnosis of upper respiratory infection. The infant's condition worsened, and she was admitted to the pediatric ICU later that night. A thorough infectious work-up was negative. She received supportive therapy and antibiotics for a week and was discharged without medications, but she continued to have a head lag. Fourteen months later, her home was evaluated when an epidemic of illegal applications of the agricultural pesticide methyl parathion in residences was recognized. Her urinary level for p-nitrophenol, a metabolite of methyl parathion, was elevated at 89 ppb (the reference range based on the National Health and Nutrition Examination Survey is 0–63 ppb) [8].

Recognizing pesticide poisonings in children

Acute intoxications in children frequently are misdiagnosed, despite being linked closely in time with generally high exposures [9,10]. Associating low-level exposures with health consequences that manifest days, weeks, months, or years later is particularly challenging. The pediatrician plays a critical role in recognizing and preventing both poisonings and chronic health effects. Without recognition, opportunities to remove the child and other affected individuals from exposure are missed, appropriate diagnosis and treatment is compromised, and chronic sequelae may develop. In the case described, analysis of blood samples for plasma pseudocholinesterase and red blood cell acetylcholinesterase inhibition would have ensured timely diagnosis of organophosphate toxicity and allowed prompt administration of atropine sulfate and pralidoxime as an antidote (Table 1). Many other affected individuals also could have been diagnosed and treated appropriately. In many states, physicians are mandated to report suspected pesticide-related incidents in an effort to recognize epidemics and identify hazards for targeted prevention strategies (Box 1).

An environmental exposure history is required to raise the index of suspicion and to clarify the relevance of pesticides to patient health. Evaluating exposures through questions about pesticide use helps establish the role of pesticides during "sick visits" and also provides anticipatory guidance. During well-child examinations, questions about pesticide use in and around the home, at the child's school, and at the parent's workplace provide an opportunity for and indicate the appropriateness of anticipatory guidance on safe practices and prevention. When pesticide exposure is suspected in an illness or symptomatic complaint, the environmental history elicits which pesticides might be involved and the type and extent of exposure. This information provides a context for assessing whether the toxicity of the product, the exposure scenario, and the likely dose support the need for consideration of specific evaluation and treatment versus reassurance. In some cases, specialty consultation with a clinical toxicologist or occupational/ environmental medicine specialist is required (see Box 1).

In addition to developing an index of suspicion, it is helpful to recognize the main pesticide groups or chemical classes and to understand their common toxicity characteristics and management (see Table 1). Pesticides can be classified in several ways. Categorization may reflect their intended use (eg, as insecticides, fungicides, herbicides, and rodenticides, among others). These classifications have little toxicologic significance but are important to understand because consumers and manufacturers classify products in this way. Pesticides also can be classified according to their chemical class (eg, as organophosphates, N-methyl carbamates, pyrethroids, triazines, and superwarfarins). These categories are meaningful toxicologically but may not be readily apparent from product name, label, or usage category. The product label itself includes the brand name and the active ingredient (the ingredient that kills the pest). There are readily available resources that can help with identification of chemical class or toxicity based on active ingredients (see Box 1).

The common presenting symptoms and some key features of clinical evaluation and management of poisoning for pesticides commonly used in the home and garden, on pets, or applied directly to children are provided in Table 1. For symptomatic pesticide illness among young children reported to the Poison Control network, the insecticides, particularly organophosphates, pyrethrin/pyrethroids, and the repellent n,n-diethyl-m-toluamide (DEET), followed by rodenticides (long-acting superwarfarin), are most frequently represented. Borates/boric acid and carbamate insecticides also

Table 1
Acute signs and symptoms and clinical evaluation considerations for common household and garden pesticides by chemical class

Agent	Acute signs and symptoms	Clinical evaluation considerations
Insecticides		
Organophosphates (examples of active ingredients: malathion, tetrachlorvinphos, tribufos [DEF], dichlorvos [DDVP], acephate, dimethoate, ethoprop, fenitrothion, fenthion, naled, terbufos, chlorpyrifos [Dursban][a], diazinon[b])	Headache Excess salivation Lacrimation Muscle twitching Nausea Diarrhea Respiratory depression Seizures Hypotonia CNS depression Miosis	Diagnostic testing: Plasma pseudocholinesterase Red blood cell cholinesterase Certain organophosphates selectively inhibit one or the other of these enzymes. The plasma enzyme effects generally persist days to weeks; the red blood cell enzyme effects last 1 to 3 months. Consider repeat testing 3 months after exposure to determine individual nonexposed baseline. Urinary alkyl phosphates are useful up to 48 hours after exposure to document exposure. Clinical interpretation of concentrations is unknown. Neuropsychologic testing has identified persistent sequelae in some adults after acute poisoning. Treatment: Atropine sulfate Pralidoxime
N-methyl carbamates (examples of active ingredients: carbaryl [Sevin], propoxur [Baygon])	Similar to organophosphates	Diagnostic testing: Plasma pseudocholinesterase Red blood cell cholinesterase The inhibition of these enzymes by carbamates is rapidly reversible, making these less reliable for diagnostic purposes (false negative) Treatment: Atropine sulfate
Pyrethrins/pyrethroids (examples of active ingredients: permethrin, bifenthrin, cyfluthrin, cypermethrin, deltamethrin, esfenvalerate)	Allergic reactions (dermatitis, asthma, rhinitis)	Diagnostic testing: None available Treatment:

	Paresthesias (stinging, burning, itching, tingling, numbness) Facial sensations Headache Fatigue Salivation Nausea and vomiting Tremor Diarrhea Irritability Seizures	Symptomatic treatment (eg. antihistamines, topical corticosteroids). Vitamin E oils are effective in preventing and stopping the paresthetic reaction
Diethyltoluamide (DEET)	Headache Restlessness Irritability Ataxia Loss of consciousness Hypotension Seizures	Diagnosis: Methods for measuring blood concentrations and urinary metabolites are not widely available
Boric acid	Mucous membrane irritation and dryness Cough Shortness of breath Beefy red skin rash on palms soles, buttocks, scrotum Nausea Diarrhea Hypothermia	Diagnosis: Urine or serum levels can be measured for confirmation

(continued on next page)

Table 1 (*continued*)

Agent	Acute signs and symptoms	Clinical evaluation considerations
Herbicides		
Chlorphenoxy compounds (examples of active ingredients: 2,4-dichorophenoxyacetic acid (2,4-D), mecoprop, dicamba)	Mucous membrane irritant Skin irritant Vomiting Diarrhea Headache Confusion Bizarre or aggressive behavior Myotonia, muscle weakness Peculiar odor on breath Metabolic acidosis, renal failure	Diagnosis: Urine concentrations can confirm overexposure (must be collected immediately; complete excretion occurs within 24–72 hours) Electromyographic and nerve conduction velocities in recovering adult patients have demonstrated mild proximal neuropathy and myopathy that persists months after acute poisoning Treatment: Alkaline diuresis in severe poisonings
Phosphonates (active ingredient: glyphosate [Roundup, Glyfonox])	Mucous membrane irritation Skin irritant	—
Rodenticides		
Coumarins and indadiones (examples of active ingredients: brodifacoum, warfarin, bromadiolone, coumachlor, coumatetralyl, difenacoum, chlorophacinone, diphacinone, pivalyn)	Bleeding/bruising (gum, nose) Fatigue Dyspnea on exertion	Diagnosis: Prothrombin time at 24 and 48 hours (Occurs within 24–48 hours of ingestion and persists 1–3 weeks) Treatment: None if certain no more than mouthful of treated bait was ingested Vitamin K1 (phytonadione) if prothrombin time is elevated or there are clinical signs of bleeding

Abbreviation: CNS, central nervous symptoms.

[a] Sale of products for indoor use banned in 2001.

[b] Sale of products for indoor use banned in 2002.

Box 1. Additional resources for pediatricians addressing pesticide toxicity concerns

Determining the types of pesticide ingredients/chemicals in specific products

The National Library of Medicine's Household Products Database provides a readily available interface to identify product ingredients based on product brand names at http://hpd.nlm.nih.gov/.

A treating physician can obtain the full list of product ingredients (including inert ingredients) directly from the company by calling the telephone number listed on the product label. To obtain this information, the physician may be required to sign a confidentiality agreement.

Once the list of ingredients is available, the chemical class can be obtained from various sources. The Pesticide Action Network database on pesticide exposures, symptoms, and toxicity (http://www.pesticideinfo.org) provides information on chemical class, covers both acute and chronic health effects, and is especially useful for agricultural exposures.

Clinical information on acute exposure signs and symptoms and recommended diagnostic and treatment strategies for specific pesticides

The EPA's *Handbook Recognition and Management of Pesticide Poisonings* covers toxicology, signs and symptoms of poisoning, and treatment of the major types of pesticides. The most recent fifth edition (1999) is available in Spanish, English, and on the Web (http://www.epa.gov/pesticides/safety/healthcare/handbook/handbook.htm).

Regional Poison Control Centers and their affiliated clinical toxicologists can be reached at 1-800-222-1222.

Information about chronic exposure to specific pesticides and other professional consultation on pesticide toxicity

The National Pesticide Medical Monitoring Program (NPMMP) is a cooperative agreement between Oregon State University and the United States Environmental Protection Agency. The NPMMP provides informational assistance in the assessment of human exposure to pesticides by e-mail (npmmp@oregonstate.edu) or by fax at (541) 737-9047.

The Pediatric Environmental Health Specialty Units are coordinated by the Association of Occupational and Environmental Clinics to provide regional academically based free consultation for health care providers. Funding is provided by the EPA and the Agency for Toxic Substances and Disease Registry (ATSDR). The Web site is http://www.aoec.org/PEHSU.htm. The toll-free telephone number is (888) 347-AOEC (2632).

Pesticide incident reporting requirements for health care providers
Contact the State Health Department

Analytical laboratories for pesticides in blood and urine
The NPMMP is affiliated with the Centers for Disease Control and provides quantitative laboratory measurements of pesticides in environmental or biologic samples in select cases involving human exposure to pesticides
For identification of commercial laboratories capable of nonroutine analyses for pesticides and metabolites, contact the regional Poison Control Center or regional Pediatric Environmental Health Specialty Unit.

Patient information on pest-control alternatives, safe use of pesticides
The EPA publication, *Citizens Guide to Pest Control and Pesticide Safety*, teaches consumers how to control pests in and around the home, alternatives to chemical pesticides, how to choose pesticides, and how to use, store, and dispose of them safely. It also discusses how to reduce exposure when others use pesticides, how to prevent pesticide poisoning and how to handle an emergency, how to choose a pest-control company, and what to do if someone is poisoned by a pesticide. (2.4 MB, available at http://www.epa.gov/OPPTpubs/Cit_Guide/citguide.pdf.)
The University of California maintains a Web site on integrated pest-management approaches for common home and garden pests. (Available at http://www.ipm.ucdavis.edu/.)

Workplace health and safety information
Information on the EPA worker protection standards is available at http://www.epa.gov/pesticides/health/worker.htm.
Employee fact sheets developed by the State of California Worker Health and Safety Branch are available at http://www.cdpr.ca.gov/docs/whs/psisenglish.htm.

Other resources
The National Library of Medicine has a comprehensive and well-organized list of Web link resources on pesticides. It can be accessed at http://sis.nlm.nih.gov/enviro/pesticides.html.

constitute a large proportion of reports to poison centers. The following sections discuss some of the common exposure issues encountered in general pediatric practice.

Organophosphates

In the case of organophosphate poisoning presented previously, the classic symptoms of cholinergic excess from the inhibition of acetylcholinesterase were not apparent. Medical students, clinical toxicologists, and emergency room physicians often are taught acronyms for the constellation of symptoms reflecting this toxicologic mechanism. One example is M-U-D-D-L-E-S: miosis, urination, diarrhea, diaphoresis, lacrimation, excitation of the central nervous system, and salivation. This acronym works reasonably well in adults. Reviews of case series, however, indicate that pediatric organophosphate poisonings often manifest with hypotonia or changes in mental status such as lethargy and coma, as well as seizures, the last being relatively rare in adult organophosphate poisoning [11]. The nonspecific symptoms of acute pesticide toxicity are easily attributed to common pediatric diagnoses such as respiratory infections, viral syndromes, gastroenteritis, atopic dermatitis, or drug-related encephalopathy. This differential underscores the importance of questions about pesticide in a thorough pediatric exposure history.

n,n-Diethyl-m-toluamide

Although technically DEET is a repellent, not a pesticide, it is discussed here because it is used against pests and is recommended by the Centers for Disease Control and Prevention and the American Academy of Pediatrics (AAP) as a strategy for prevention of mosquito-borne disease such as West Nile encephalitis [12,13]. Although rare, there have been reports of severe neurotoxicity associated with exposure to DEET; therefore the AAP recommends precautions when this product is used on children [14–16]. For example, using lower concentrations of DEET products (preferably 10% and no more than 30%), avoiding formulations containing ethanol or permethrin, and using the product only on intact, uncovered skin will reduce the dermally absorbed dose. Infants less than 2 months of age have increased dermal absorption, so use in this population is not recommended. In addition, products containing mixtures of DEET and sunscreen should be avoided, because sunscreen may require reapplication for effectiveness, and no more than a single daily application of DEET is recommended.

Scabicides and pediculocides

Permethrin and malathion, and in some cases lindane, may be used as topically applied insecticides to treat lice and scabies. The potential toxicity of malathion and its flammable alcohol base make it undesirable. Lindane has been associated with significant neurotoxicity, and the AAP recommends its cautious use as a second-line agent in select populations of older children [17]. Its use has been banned entirely in some states and in numerous other countries because of the potential for serious water contamination, environmental toxicity, and long-term environmental persistence [18]. The pyrethrin/pyrethroid-containing products have been used extensively with limited adverse events reports. There is an adult case report of an anaphylactoid reaction after use of a pyrethrin-containing shampoo and a case of a fatal asthma death occurred in a child after she applied a pyrethrin-based animal shampoo on a pet [19,20]. Although the process is labor intensive, head lice in children can be managed effectively and safely with repeated combing of hair and washing of clothing and bedding in hot water.

Residential products

Following recent bans on chlorpyrifos and diazinon (both organophosphates) for residential use, the household insecticides now in common use contain other organophosphates (malathion, tetrachlorvinphos, dichlorvos), N-methyl carbamates (carbaryl, propoxur), and, increasingly, pyrethroids/pyrethrins, or combinations. Broadcast applications, including sprays, "flea bombs," and foggers are more problematic than spot or crack and crevice applications; the latter methods, in turn, can be replaced safely in many situations by enclosed insect baits or traps. After spraying, insecticide residues can linger on the floor, in the air, in carpets, on toys, and in the dust [21,22]. Children crawling on these surfaces and putting their hands or objects in their mouths can ingest significant quantities of pesticides [23]. The vapor of some pesticide sprays lingers near ground level, in the breathing zone of a toddler [24]. Even lawn and garden herbicides can be tracked in to homes, especially homes where a dog uses the back yard, and can linger in carpets, resulting in potentially significant child exposures [25].

The symptomatic complaints related to pyrethrin/pyrethroids are often skin related (stinging, burning, itching, tingling, numbness, paresthesias), and these agents have been associated with contact dermatitis and allergic respiratory reaction (rhinitis, asthma) [11]. Their other signs and symptoms overlap with the nonspecific nature of organophosphate overexposure (see Table 1).

For most household pest problems (as well as lawn and garden uses), less toxic alternatives and integrated pest-management approaches can be employed and should be encouraged (see Box 1). In particular, insecticides can be replaced by an approach that includes cleaning up food and water, sealing cracks and crevices, and using pesticides that are contained in baits or traps, which are far less likely to pose a health concern compared with any type of spray application. Lawns and gardens can be maintained by avoiding combination products with pesticides and fertilizers (ie, "weed and feed" preparations) that tend to result in overapplication of pesticides. Hand weeding is always a reasonable alternative to herbicides. If herbicides are used, some (such as glyphosate) have far better toxicity profiles than others (such as 2,4-dichlorophenoxyacetic acid). Parents also should be advised regarding proper storage of pesticides (in a locked cabinet or building) and against reuse of pesticide containers.

As sold to consumers, pesticide products contain a mixture of active ingredients (usually one or two) and a variety of other ingredients (sometimes called "inert" ingredients). The concentration of the active ingredient varies widely from one product to another; for example, DEET formulations range from 10% to 100%, and the concentration of permethrin products can range from 0.02% to 99.5%. Inert ingredients include solvents, emulsifiers, diluents, stabilizers, adjuvants, and even fragrances. Any ingredient that does not kill the pest is considered an inert ingredient. Inert ingredients are listed on the label as "other ingredients" and are not named specifically. Generally the other ingredients are trade secrets, and it is difficult to get any information about them. These chemicals may have their own toxicities, however, particularly as irritants to skin and mucous membranes, including the lower respiratory tract. A health care provider who is treating a patient exposed to a particular pesticide product can call the manufacturer and obtain the full list of ingredients. To do so often involves signing an agreement not to disclose the information to anyone.

Other important sources of household pesticide exposure

Occupational exposures to parent and child

Other important exposure scenarios for children include their own or parent's occupation. Adolescents may find summer employment in landscaping, pool care, or agricultural work. Although this work may be temporary or part-time in nature, adolescents may be less likely to appreciate or be informed about the risk of using chemicals in their work. In most states, a person under age 18 years cannot become a licensed pesticide applicator, although unlicensed pesticide application is common, and pesticide exposures can occur even if the child is not applying the chemical. Working parents and children may carry home exposure as residues on clothing or shoes. People who may be occupationally exposed to pesticides should understand the importance of personal protective equipment such as appropriate respirators, gloves, and coveralls, hand washing after contact with chemicals, removal of work clothes, and separate laundering of work clothes. Parents who handle pesticides at work should be careful not to come home with residues on their skin, clothes, or shoes.

Pesticides in the food supply

Dietary exposures to pesticide residues also may be important, especially because children eat a relatively restricted diet, choose certain dietary items (eg, bananas or apples) relatively frequently, and consume far larger portions on a bodyweight-adjusted basis than do adults [26]. The dietary pathway has become a significant concern relative to the organophosphate insecticides. These chemicals are used heavily on some of the fruits that are common dietary staples among children. A study in which children were placed on an organic diet for a period of 5 consecutive days revealed a rapid and dramatic drop in their urinary excretion of organophosphate metabolites [27].

High-risk populations

Pesticide exposures are not distributed evenly across the population. Children of farm workers and urban poor children may be at particular risk. In addition, individual child behaviors can have an important impact. Studies of toddlers at day care centers have demonstrate that children who are more active and interact more intimately with their environment (eg, by frequently putting objects in their mouths) receive a dermal dose of pesticide that is 600-fold greater than that of other toddlers in the same environment [28]. Children living in agricultural communities and those whose parents work in agriculture have been shown to be exposed to higher concentrations of insecticides and to excrete metabolites of pesticides that are not registered for household use in their urine [29]. Low-income households of color are more likely to use broadcast, dispersive methods of insecticidal application [30], probably reflecting the quality of the housing stock and the lack of control in making decisions about pesticide use. Housing with many cracks, moisture problems, and holes is more likely to harbor pest infestations. Similarly, living in rental housing or public housing, where landlords may engage in routine spraying, does not offer parents much opportunity to make their own decisions about pesticide use around their children.

Chronic health concerns with pesticide exposures

Fortunately, acute poisoning events in children are relatively rare. The health implications of exposures encountered routinely at low levels have become an increasing focus of concern for scientists, regulators, and communities [31,32]. Although a pediatrician may never diagnose an acute poisoning, most will be relied upon as a trusted source for questions about potential long-term or subtle health effects from pesticide residues on food, in water, or used in homes or schools.

Responding to such questions requires an exposure history to clarify the extent and types of exposures, some knowledge about the toxicity of various chemicals and outcomes, and a common-sense approach toward recommending the safest practical alternative. Helpful data may come from experimental animal models, veterinary science, and epidemiologic studies. The breadth of possibilities and evidence are beyond the scope of this article and the expected knowledge base of the primary care pediatrician. Awareness of the primary outcomes for which there is a body of suggestive epidemiological evidence—neurodevelopmental effects, childhood cancer, birth defects, and asthma—provides a useful foundation for responding to parental concerns. A brief description of the state of the evidence is provided here.

Review articles describe a number of ecologic and case-control studies that have associated parental exposures or pesticide use in the home with childhood brain tumors, leukemias and lymphomas, and a number of other tumor types [33,34]. The reader is referred to the article by Buka, Koranteng, and Vargas in this issue for more detail on the strengths and limitations of these and more recent data.

Birth defects studies have linked parental occupational pesticide exposure with cryptorchidism, orofacial clefts, limb reduction defects, and heart defects in their children [35–37]. Associations have been observed with both maternal and paternal exposures. For most of these and the pediatric cancer studies, however, the assessment of exposure is for pesticides in general rather than for specific agents or classes of agents. Thus the understanding of the associations is limited and the ability to specify prevention strategies is hampered.

In contrast, much of the evidence for neurodevelopmental effects is focused specifically on studies of organophosphate insecticide exposure. There has been a rapid emergence of evidence demonstrating the neurodevelopmental toxicity of these agents at relatively low exposure levels [38–40]. This evidence includes animal studies describing the mechanistic basis as well as emerging data from studies in the United States population. Animal studies demonstrate that the timing of exposure as well as the dose influences the toxicity manifestations, and adverse effects occur even at low exposure levels that do not affect acetylcholinesterase [41].

Epidemiologic evidence of harm to young children has been described in three large ongoing cohort studies in the United States [6,39,40]. These studies recruited pregnant women and characterized their exposure to certain organophosphates (and in some cases to other pesticides and other environmental contaminants) in pregnancy and in the newborn period using environmental measures, questionnaires, and biologic markers. The newborns were followed through infancy and early childhood to assess their neurodevelopmental health and determine if pesticide exposure in utero and early childhood has adverse effects on neurodevelopmental and behavioral function. Adverse birth outcomes also were evaluated, and respiratory health evaluations are planned as the children age.

Two of these studies are based in urban New York City. The Mt. Sinai–based Children's Environmental cohort study reported that among mothers who had detectable levels of chlorpyrifos metabolites (an organophosphate) in their urine, those with low activity of the enzyme paraoxonase (PON1), which is involved in the detoxification of chlorpyrifos, gave birth to infants with significantly reduced head circumferences compared with mothers with higher activity of PON1 [6]. The authors note that because small head size has been shown to predict subsequent cognitive ability, these data suggest that exposure to chlorpyrifos may have an adverse effect on the fetal neuro-development in offspring of mothers who have genetic risk factors (low PON1 activity).

Preliminary findings from a cohort of mothers and infants being studied by the Columbia Center for Children's Environmental Health also suggest that children who have high chlorpyrifos exposure prenatally have an increased risk of motor and cognitive development delay. In addition, among the most highly exposed, a significantly higher number of children manifested symptoms of inattention at age 3 years [39].

A study of farm workers' children in California, conducted by The Center for the Heath Assessment of Mothers and Children of Salinas, assessed infants in the first months of life using the Brazelton Neonatal Behavioral Assessment Scale (BNBAS) [40]. As maternal prenatal metabolite levels of organophosphate insecticides increased, a dose-related increase in abnormal reflexes was observed. A 10-fold increase of maternal metabolites was associated with a fivefold increase of more than three abnormal reflexes (odds ratio [OR], 4.9; 95% confidence interval [CI], 1.5–16.1). No association was observed between maternal postnatal urinary metabolite concentrations and BNBAS findings.

As these cohort studies evaluate respiratory health and asthma development in children from infancy to school age, they will augment a limited body of epidemiologic data regarding the role of pesticides in pediatric asthma and respiratory health. Existing published reports are few and mixed. An assessment of children in agricultural Iowa did not find an association between pesticide use indoors and out and increased asthma symptoms [42]. A large survey of Lebanese children, however, found that pesticide exposure in the home, pesticide exposure related to parent's occupation, and pesticide exposure outside the home were associated with an increased risk of respiratory diseases overall [43]. The highest risk was observed for children whose parents had occupational exposure to pesticides (OR, 4.61; 95% CI, 2.06–10.29). Evidence of an adverse association also is seen in a nested case-control study of children involved in the Children's Health Study of Southern California. Among environmental exposures examined in the first year of life, herbicides and pesticides had the strongest association with asthma diagnosis before age 5 years (OR, 4.58; 95% CI, 1.36–15.43 and OR, 2.39; 95% CI, 1.17–4.89, respectively) [44]. Data are accumulating from large studies that p,p′-dichlorodiphenyldichloroethylene (DDE), a metabolite of the now-banned but persistent environmental contaminant, the insecticide dichlorodiphenyltrichloroethane (DDT), may be a risk factor for asthma and elevated IgE levels [45,46].

Clearly, the state of the evidence concerning the effect of pesticide exposure on pediatric health has a number of inadequacies. Most epidemiologic studies have limited exposure assessment, so risk cannot be assessed in relation to specific pesticide types or doses. Studies are not uniform in identifying health risks. Many pesticide compounds have not been investigated for chronic health effects, in either animal models or epidemiologic designs. Nonetheless, there is a growing and improving body of suggestive evidence of harm at exposure levels that occur in United States populations. Of note, investigators have begun to explore the potential modification of risk based on genetic influences [5,6]. These approaches can reveal associations that are not apparent when the gene–environment effect is not considered.

Addressing common questions in primary care pediatrics

The pediatrician may encounter a wide range of questions from patients regarding exposures to pesticides and health risks. Examples of the nature of questions might include.

Will my daughter's attention deficit hyperactivity disorder be worsened if we use pesticides on our lawn?

Is it because my husband is a pesticide applicator that my daughter has a heart defect?

Should I buy organic food for my children?

Is my exterminator right that my 2-year-old is at no risk from flea bombing our house if I air the house out sufficiently before returning?

I have ants in the house and want to get rid of them. What's the safest way?

Although there are a variety of ways of dealing with such questions, it is helpful to have a preventive, compassionate approach as well as ideas for resources where patients may seek additional information. Questions about whether historical pesticide exposure may have caused a disease or birth defect in a child are very difficult to answer. Sometimes these questions arise in a legal context, but often they show a concern that a patient expresses simply out of an effort to make sense of an adverse event. Although it certainly is possible to establish causation of acute pesticide poisoning, it is extremely difficult to associate an historic pesticide exposure—to parents or children—with a specific adverse outcome in a child. Such questions are best addressed by a specialist in pediatric environmental health (see Box 1).

Questions regarding the safety of pesticide use in the garden and home and regarding ways to solve specific pest problems safely are extremely common. Although pesticides can be useful in certain circumstances and can be used safely, it is best to use least-toxic approaches first. In communicating this philosophy to a patient, it is helpful to clarify that although the use of pesticides will be unlikely to result in a specific health effect (such as worsening of a child's attention deficit hyperactivity disorder, as in the example given previously), pesticides are designed to be potent toxic chemicals, and a precautionary approach would advise their avoidance when possible. This method of pest control is called "integrated pest management." Some resources for integrated pest-management approaches to home and garden pest control are listed in Box 1.

Often parents want to know whether they should feed their children an organic-only diet. Organic food is a rapidly growing segment of the United States food market. It is possible to obtain organic foods in most parts of the country at most times of year, but organic foods usually are higher priced. Conventionally grown foods frequently contain pesticide residues at low concentrations, and such residues are rarely found on organic food. Children placed experimentally on an organic diet experienced a dramatic decline in organophosphate pesticide metabolites in their urine over 5 days [27]. Reviews of government residue-testing data suggest that certain foods, such as apples, bell peppers, celery, imported grapes, cherries, peaches, potatoes, pears, raspberries, spinach, and strawberries, tend to be high in pesticide residues and should be priorities for purchasing organically, whereas others, such as asparagus, avocado, bananas, broccoli, sweet corn, onions, and peas, rarely contain residues even if grown conventionally [47]. These guidelines may be useful for consumers who are concerned about pesticide residues on food but cannot afford to purchase only organically grown food for their children.

Summary

Pediatricians are a trusted source of information, can positively influence parental behavior, and can provide important anticipatory guidance regarding pesticide exposure. Both the potential for acute poisoning and concern about effects on chronic health make it essential that the pediatric care provider maintain a high index of suspicion and offer informed guidance on reduction of pesticide exposure. Anticipatory guidance to prevent direct access by children to pesticides and also to reduce the use of broadcast pesticide applications in children's environments can prevent potentially significant exposures. To address patient concerns, it is important for pediatricians to know the basic facts and have appropriate resources to turn to for answers.

References

[1] Whitmore RW, Kelly JE, Reading PL. The national home and garden pesticide survey. vol. 1. Executive summary, results, and recommendations. Prepared by Research Triangle Institute. Rpt no RTI/5100/17–01F. Washington, DC: U.S. Environmental Protection Agency; 1992.

[2] Committee on Pesticides in the Diets of Infants and Children. Pesticides in the diets of infants and children. Washington, DC: National Academies Press; 1993. Available at: http://www.nap.edu/catalog/2126.html. Accessed January 15, 2007.

[3] Faustman EM, Silbernagel SM, Fenske RA, et al. Mechanisms underlying children's susceptibility to environmental toxicants. Environ Health Perspect 2000;108(Suppl 1):13–21.

[4] Bradman A, Whyatt RM. Characterizing exposures to non persistent pesticides during pregnancy and early childhood in the national children's study: a review of monitoring and measurement methodologies. Environ Health Perspect 2005;113:1092–9.

[5] Nielsen SS, Mueller BA, DeRoos AJ, et al. Risk of brain tumors in children and susceptibility to organophosphorus insecticides: the potential role of paraoxonase (PON1). Environ Health Perspect 2005;113:909–13.

[6] Berkowitz GS, Wetmur JG, Birman-Deych E, et al. In utero pesticide exposure, maternal paraoxonase activity, and head circumference. Environ Health Perspect 2004;112:388–9.

[7] National Center for Environmental Health Division of Laboratory Sciences. National Report on Human Exposure to Environmental Chemicals. Atlanta, GA: Centers for Disease Control and Prevention; 2005. NCEH Pub. No. 05-0570. http://www.cdc.gov/exposurereport/.

[8] Rubin C, Esteban E, Kieszak S, et al. Assessment of human exposure and human health effects after indoor application of methyl parathion in Lorain County, Ohio, 1995-1996. Environ Health Perspect 2002;110(Suppl 6):1047–51.

[9] Zwiener RJ, Ginsburg CM. Organophosphate and carbamate poisoning in infants and children [published erratum appears in Pediatrics 1988 May;81(5):683]. Pediatrics 1988;81:121–6.

[10] Sopher S, Tal A, Shahak E. Carbamate and organophosphate poisoning in early childhood. Pediatr Emerg Care 1989;5:222–5.

[11] Reigart JR, Roberts JR. Recognition and management of pesticide poisonings. Fifth edition. Washington, DC: U.S. EPA; 1999.

[12] Kiely T, Donaldson D, Grube A. Pesticide industry sales and usage: 2000–2001 market estimates. U.S. Environmental Protection Agency, Washington, DC. May 2004.

[13] American Academy of Pediatrics Committee on Infectious Diseases. Prevention of lyme disease. Pediatrics 2000;105(1):142–7.

[14] Osimitz TG, Murphy JV. Neurological effects associated with use of the insect repellent N,N-diethyl-m-toluamide (DEET). J Toxicol Clin Toxicol 1997;35(5):435–41.

[15] Sudakin DL, Trevathan WR. DEET: a review and update of safety and risk in the general population. J Toxicol Clin Toxicol 2003;41(6):831–9.

[16] American Academy of Pediatrics Committee on Environmental Health. Follow safety precautions when using DEET on children. AAP News 2003;22:99.

[17] Frankowski BL, Weiner LB. Committee on School Health the Committee on Infectious Diseases. American Academy of Pediatrics. Head lice. Pediatrics 2002;110:638–43.

[18] Frankowski BL. American Academy of Pediatrics guidelines for the prevention and treatment of head lice infestation. Am J Manag Care 2004;10(9 Suppl):S269–72.

[19] Culver CA, Malina JJ, Talbert RL. Probable anaphylactoid reaction to a pyrethrin pediculocide shampoo. Clin Pharm 1988;7:846–9.

[20] Wagner SL. Fatal asthma in a child after use of an animal shampoo containing pyrethrin. West J Med 2000;173(2):86–7.

[21] Lewis RG, Fortune CR, Blanchard FT, et al. Movement and deposition of two organophosphorus pesticides within a residence after interior and exterior applications. J Air Waste Manag Assoc 2001;51(3):339–51.

[22] Hore P, Robson M, Freeman N, et al. Chlorpyrifos accumulation patterns for child-accessible surfaces and objects and urinary metabolite excretion by children for 2 weeks after crack-and-crevice application. Environ Health Perspect 2005;113:211–9.

[23] Gurunathan S, Robson M, Freeman N, et al. Accumulation of chlorpyrifos on residential surfaces and toys accessible to children. Environ Health Perspect 1998;106(1):9–16.

[24] Fenske RA, Black KG, Elkner KP, et al. Potential exposure and health risks of infants following indoor residential pesticide applications. Am J Public Health 1990;80(6):689–93.

[25] Nishioka MG, Lewis RG, Brinkman MC, et al. Distribution of 2,4-D in air and on surfaces inside residences after lawn applications: comparing exposure estimates from various media for young children. Environ Health Perspect 2001;109(11):1185–91.

[26] Selevan SG, Kimmel CA, Mendola P. Identifying critical windows of exposure for children's health. Environ Health Perspect 2000;108(suppl 3):451–5.

[27] Lu C, Toepel K, Irish R, et al. Organic diets significantly lower children's dietary exposure to organophosphorus pesticides. Environ Health Perspect 2006;114(2):260–3.

[28] Cohen Hubal EA, Egeghy PP, Leovic KW, et al. Measuring potential dermal transfer of a pesticide to children in a child care center. Environ Health Perspect 2006;114(2): 264–9.

[29] Lu C, Fenske RA, Simcox NJ, et al. Pesticide exposure of children in an agricultural community: evidence of household proximity to farmland and take home exposure pathways. Environ Res 2000;84(3):290–302.

[30] McKelvey W, Kass D, Sorkin M, et al. Early reports from an urban pesticide tracking system: the use and misuse of pesticides in New York City. New York: Department of Health and Mental Hygiene; 2005.

[31] U.S. Environmental Protection Agency. Food Quality Protection Act of 1996. (P.L. 104-170).

[32] National Institute of Environmental Health Sciences. Children's Environmental Health Research Centers Press Release August 10, 1998 (#15–98). Available at: http://www.niehs.nih.gov/oc/news/niehsepa.htm. Accessed January 15, 2007.

[33] Daniels JL, Olshan AF, Savitz DA. Pesticides and childhood cancers. Environ Health Perspect 1997;105(10):1068–77.

[34] Zahm SH, Devesa SS. Childhood cancer: overview of incidence trends and environmental carcinogens. Environ Health Perspec 1995;103(Suppl 3):177–84.

[35] Hanke W, Jurewicz J. The risk of adverse reproductive and developmental disorders due to occupational pesticide exposure: an overview of current epidemiological evidence. Int J Occup Med Environ Health 2004;17:223–43.

[36] Garcia AM. Occupational exposure to pesticides and congenital malformations: a review of mechanisms, methods, and results. Am J Ind Med 1998;33:232–40.

[37] Shaw GM, Wasserman CR, O'Malley CD, et al. Maternal pesticide exposure from multiple sources and selected congenital anomalies. Epidemiology 1999;10:60–6.

[38] Slotkin TA. Cholinergic systems in brain development and disruption by neurotoxicants: nicotine, environmental tobacco smoke, organophosphates. Toxicol Appl Pharmacol 2004;198:132–51.

[39] Rauh VA, Garfinkel R, Perera FP, et al. Impact of prenatal chlorpyrifos exposure on neurodevelopment in the first 3 years of life among inner-city children. Pediatrics 2006;118: e1845–59.

[40] Young JG, Eskenazi B, Gladstone EA, et al. Association between in utero organophosphate pesticide exposure and abnormal reflexes in neonates. NeuroToxicology 2005;26:199–209.

[41] Slotkin TA. Guidelines for developmental neurotoxicity and their impact on organophosphate pesticides: a personal view from an academic perspective. Neurotoxicology 2004; 25(4):631–40.

[42] Merchant JA, Naleway AL, Svendsen ER, et al. Asthma and farm exposures in a cohort of rural Iowa children. Environ Health Perspect 2005;113:350–6.

[43] Salameh PR, Baldi I, Brochard P, et al. Respiratory symptoms in children and exposure to pesticides. Eur Respir J 2003;22:507–12.

[44] Salam MT, Yu-Fen L, Langholz B, et al. Early life environmental risk factors for asthma: findings from the children's health study. Environ Health Perspect 2004;112:760–5.

[45] Karmaus W, Kruse H. Infections and atopic disorders in childhood and organochlorine exposure. Arch Env Health 2001;56:485–92.

[46] Sunyer J, Torrent M, Muñoz-Ortiz L, et al. Prenatal dichlorodiphenyldichloroethylene (DDE) and asthma in children. Environ Health Perspect 2005;113:1787–90.

[47] Environmental Working Group. Shoppers guide to pesticides in produce. Washington, DC. Available at: http://www.foodnews.org/walletguide.php. Accessed June 10, 2006.

PEDIATRIC CLINICS
OF NORTH AMERICA

Pediatr Clin N Am
54 (2007) 81–101

Transgenerational Exposures: Persistent Chemical Pollutants in the Environment and Breast Milk

Josef G. Thundiyil, MD, MPH[a,b,c],
Gina M. Solomon, MD, MPH[b,d,e],
Mark D. Miller, MD, MPH[e,*]

[a]California Poison Control System, University of California-San Francisco,
San Francisco, CA, USA
[b]Division of Occupational and Environmental Medicine,
University of California-San Francisco, San Francisco, CA, USA
[c]Department of Emergency Medicine, Orlando Regional Medical Center,
Orlando, FL, USA
[d]Natural Resources Defense Council, San Francisco, CA, USA
[e]UCSF Pediatric Environmental Health Specialty Unit, California Poison Control System,
University of California-San Francisco, San Francisco, CA, USA

Many environmental threats to children's health are chemicals or pollutants that are currently used or released into the environment, such as pesticides, mercury, various chemicals in consumer products, and air pollutants. Some chemicals, however, remain significant health concerns even though they have been banned for more than a quarter-century in the United States. Many of these so-called "legacy pollutants" are also known as "persistent organic pollutants" (POPs). These substances are present within the food supply, and they are known to accumulate in breast milk. Because many POPs, such as dichlorodiphenyltrichlorethane (DDT), polychlorinated biphenyls (PCBs), and dioxins, are familiar names, there is a high level of concern among the general public about these contaminants. In addition, sporadic media attention about contaminants in food and breast milk

The University of California Pediatric Environmental Health Specialty Unit receives funding from the US Agency for Toxic Substances Disease Registry and the US Environmental Protection Agency administered by the Association of Occupational and Environmental Clinics.

* Corresponding author.
E-mail address: mmiller@oehha.ca.gov (M.D. Miller).

generates questions to pediatricians about the likelihood and nature of potential health effects and about the advisability of breastfeeding.

POPs are synthetic organic compounds that persist in the environment for many years, resist biodegradation, accumulate in fatty tissues and in predator species, and travel long distances to be dispersed globally. Nearly all living organisms carry measurable concentrations of POPs in their bodies [1]. Although POP chemicals have a variety of structural characteristics, most are polyaromatic, and all are polyhalogenated hydrocarbons, usually containing chlorine or bromine as an important constituent. A dozen POPs have been targeted for global elimination under the Stockholm Convention on Persistent Organic Pollutants [2], an international treaty signed by 151 countries in May, 2001. The pesticides and industrial chemicals on the Stockholm POPs list were banned in most developed countries in the late 1970s, although many are still in use in the developing world. Other chemicals that share POPs' characteristics remain in widespread use in the United States and worldwide.

Extensive human cohort studies have shown associations between certain POPs, particularly PCBs and dioxins, and a wide array of adverse health effects in infants and children. Although the health effects generally are subtle, they are of significant concern because they have been shown to occur at exposure concentrations within the range commonly found in the human population worldwide. Epidemiologic studies have demonstrated adverse neurodevelopmental effects [3–10], endocrine alterations [11–20], immunotoxicity [21–28], and increased cancer risk [29–32] in populations with above-average exposures to these chemicals.

Persistence and bioaccumulation

An important characteristic of POPs is their ability to resist photolytic, biologic, and chemical degradation. They have half-lives that range from months to more than a decade. These chemicals are semivolatile, which allows them to evaporate into the atmosphere and deposit back to earth in precipitation. As this cycle is repeated, these substances are transported from equatorial regions toward the poles in a process called "global distillation" [33]. This process accounts for the high concentrations of POPs in Arctic wildlife [34]. POPs are also lipophilic and hydrophobic [2]. When these chemicals land in water, they precipitate rapidly from the water column and attach to organic material in the sediment, where they may be consumed by small organisms.

As organisms at the bottom of the food chain consume POPs, these substances are absorbed and stored in fatty tissue. Because POPs are not readily excreted, continued consumption over time results in bioconcentration. As higher-level predators consume lower-level organisms, the increasing concentration is accentuated in a process referred to as "biomagnification." This phenomenon holds particularly true for aquatic ecosystems because there are more levels in the food chain. Native peoples in the Arctic regions derive a substantial portion of their diet from high on the food chain (ie, marine mammals); they are among the populations most highly exposed to POPs.

Breastfeeding infants are at the top of the food chain, and they consume bioaccumulated substances in mother's milk [35]. Infants are at additional risk because of their relatively high adipose concentrations, rapidly developing organs, and high intake of food or breast milk relative to body weight.

Sources

Diet is the major predictor for POPs exposures [36]. Although fruits, vegetables, and grains contain small amounts of POPs, the highest exposure comes from consumption of animal fats. Fig. 1 summarizes the main sources of dietary intake of dioxin for various age groups of children.

POPs are known to occur in human breast milk. Concentrations of various POPs are up to six times higher in breast milk than in maternal serum, and it has been estimated that infants breastfeeding for 6 months may receive as much as 14% of their cumulative lifetime exposure of dioxins and PCBs [37]. Because of the prolonged half-life of dioxin, this childhood exposure contributes significantly to the total body burden present during the

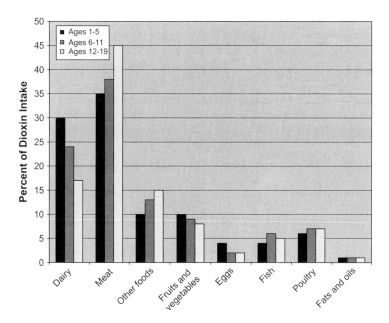

Fig. 1. Estimated percent contribution of various foods to dioxin intake among children. (*Data from* The Committee on the Implications of Dioxin in the Food Supply. Dioxins and dioxin-like compounds in the food supply: strategies to decrease exposure. Washington, DC: National Academies Press; 2003. p. 116–20.)

reproductive years. Fortunately, the concentrations of most POPs in breast milk have shown a significant decline in the past few decades as a result of increasing restrictions on production and use worldwide. Fig. 2 illustrates the decline of several major POPs in breast milk. The World Health Organization and the American Academy of Pediatrics have concluded that the health benefits of breastfeeding are not outweighed by the presence of pollutants [38,39].

Persistent organic pollutants controlled under international treaty

The Stockholm Convention on Persistent Organic Pollutants was signed by 151 countries, including the United States [2]. Its goal is to eliminate or restrict the use of 12 major POPs (Table 1). Additional chemicals have been nominated to join these original 12. Although the United States has not ratified the Stockholm Convention, most of these chemicals have been banned in the United States for many years. These chemicals can be classified generally into three major categories: pesticides, industrial chemicals, and byproducts.

Nine of the 12 Stockholm POPs were used as pesticides for vector control and agriculture. These chemicals came into widespread use after World War Two and initially had the advantage of minimal acute toxicity. Concerns about persistence and chronic toxicity led many countries to ban their use in the 1970s. Some of pesticides banned by the Stockholm Convention, such as DDT, are still used for vector control in developing countries.

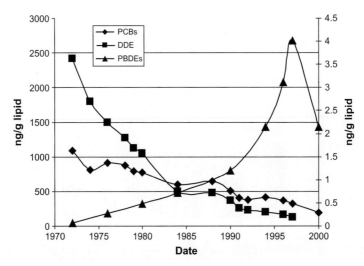

Fig. 2. Time trends of representative persistent organic pollutants in human breast milk. DDE, dicholorodiphenyldicholoroethylne; PCBs, polychlorinated biphenyls; PBDEs, polybrominated diphenyl ethers. (*Data from* Meironyte NK. Certain organochlorine and organobromine contaminants in Swedish breast milk in perspective of past 20–30 years. Chemosphere 2000;40(9–11):1111–23.)

Table 1
Persistent organic pollutants (POPs) subject to the Stockholm convention

Chemical	Category	Sources	Potential health effects	Half-life	California carcinogen classification
Aldrin	Insecticide	Agriculture, food	Neurotoxic, immune	5 years (soil)	Yes
Chlordane	Insecticide	Termite, agriculture, food	Neurotoxic, liver, immune	1 year (soil)	Yes
DDT	Insecticide	Vector control, agriculture, food	Lactation, liver, development, reproduction	10–15 years (soil)	Yes
Dieldrin	Insecticide (metabolite of Aldrin)	Agriculture, food, termite control	Neurotoxic, immune	5 years (soil)	Yes
Dioxins	Incineration byproduct	Food, waste sites	Development, immune, endocrine	7 years (humans); 10–12 years (soil)	Yes
Furans	Byproduct contaminant	Food, waste sites	As dioxin above	10–12 years (soil)	Yes
Endrin	Insecticide	Agriculture, food	Neurotoxic, development	12 years (soil)	No
Heptachlor	Insecticide	Fire ants, termite, agriculture, food	Development, neurologic, reproductive	2 years (soil)	Yes
Hexachlorobenzene	Fungicide, industrial by product	Agriculture, food	Liver, immune, endocrine	3–6 years (soil)	Yes
Mirex	Insecticide	Fire ants, termite, agriculture, food	Liver, neurologic, reproductive	10 years (sediment)	Yes
PCBs	Industrial Chemical	Food, leaking transformers, waste sites	Neurologic, development, immune, endocrine	2–6 years	Yes
Toxaphene	Insecticide	Agriculture, food	Immune, development	12 years (soil)	Yes

PCBs are halogenated hydrocarbons with paired phenyl rings having varying degrees of chlorination. Billions of pounds of these chemicals were produced for use in capacitors, transformers, and carbonless copy paper because of their fire-resistant properties [40]. In 1978 these products were banned in the United States and in many other countries, but they are still detectable in human tissue. Dioxins and furans are byproducts of combustion, waste incineration, paper bleaching, and chlorine production. There are hundreds of potential congeners, the most potent of which is 2,3,7,8-tetrachlorodibenzodioxin (TCDD). This substance has an estimated half-life in the human body of up to 7 years [41] and sometimes is referred to as the most toxic synthetic chemical known to man. Although pollution controls have reduced these chemicals, there is still ongoing release into the environment.

Human health effects of banned persistent organic pollutants

Neurodevelopmental effects

A variety of sources have presented compelling evidence of the impact of PCBs and dioxin on children's neurodevelopment. Animal research has demonstrated negative effects of in utero PCB exposure on neurodevelopment, cerebellar functioning, and short-term memory [42]. In a cohort of humans exposed prenatally to a mass poisoning from PCB-contaminated rice oil in Taiwan, exposed children demonstrated developmental delays, behavioral abnormalities, and poor cognitive development lasting past age 11 years, as well as dermatologic effects including hyperpigmentation of the skin and nails [43].

Several prospective cohort studies have demonstrated adverse developmental and neurodevelopmental findings at significantly lower exposures typical of fish-eating populations from the Netherlands, Michigan, North Carolina, and New York. An ongoing study in the Netherlands recruited mothers during pregnancy and followed the development of their children. The researchers estimated prenatal PCB exposure based on levels in maternal plasma during the last month of pregnancy; and postnatal exposure to PCBs and dioxin was based on levels in breast milk samples and duration of breastfeeding. At birth, the more exposed children had statistically significantly smaller head circumference [44]; by age 3 months, psychomotor and neurologic development was negatively associated with prenatal PCB exposure [45]. At age 7 months, although the breastfed infants were doing better by neurologic measures than the formula-fed infants, those exposed to higher concentrations of PCBs and dioxins in the breast milk were behind their breastfed peers. Additionally, General Cognitive Index and memory scores on the McCarthy Scales of Children's Abilities remained impaired by 8% ($P < .01$) at 7 years of age among those children who had highest PCB and dioxin exposures and whose home environment was rated "less advantageous" [3].

Cohorts of children whose mothers ate fish from the Great Lakes have been followed for years in New York and Michigan. Higher in utero exposures to PCBs as measured in maternal serum and cord blood were associated with significantly smaller head circumference, lower birth weight (by an average of 180 g) [4], poorer neonatal neurologic scores [5], poorer visual recognition memory on the Fagan Test of Infant Intelligence at ages 6 and 12 months [6], and persistent cognitive deficits in verbal and numeric memory at 4 years [7]. Further, at age 11 years, the children with the highest prenatal exposure were found to have a 6.2-point decrement in IQ scores and delayed reading abilities [8]. These children were three times more likely to have low-average IQ scores and twice as likely to be at least 2 years behind in reading comprehension. Another prospective cohort study in North Carolina found that infants exposed to higher in utero PCB concentrations were significantly more likely to be hyporeflexive [9] and had seven-point lower scores, on average, on the psychomotor section of the Bayley Scales of Infant Development up to 24 months of age but had no detectable cognitive deficits at 5 years [10].

Overall, the results of these studies and others suggest that exposures to PCBs and dioxins that are only slightly higher than the average exposure in the general population may have a long-term impact on cognitive function in children. Although some studies also have pointed to an association between breast-milk levels and negative newborn neurologic scores, the breast-milk levels may represent markers for in utero exposure; these studies also indicate that breastfed infants did better than formula-fed infants regardless of the presence of PCBs and dioxins in the breast milk. The exact mechanism by which PCBs or dioxins may cause long-term cognitive impairment is unclear. The leading hypothesis points to the role of PCBs and some of the dioxins in disrupting normal thyroid function. The regulatory role of thyroid hormones on brain development has long been recognized [46]. Other factors, including incomplete development of the blood–brain barrier, lack of detoxification systems within the fetus, and the sensitivity of migratory cells undergoing mitosis, may play a role.

In a recent study conducted in the United States, prenatal exposure to DDT was associated with neurodevelopmental delays in early childhood [47]. The mothers were immigrants from Mexico and had substantially higher exposures than women born in the United States. Decreases in the Mental Development Index scores corresponding to 7 to 10 points across the exposure range were found. Breastfeeding was found to be beneficial even among highly exposed women.

Endocrine effects

Many POPs have developed notoriety for being "endocrine disruptors." The similarity of their structure to many hormones, including thyroid hormone, can, depending on the dose and congener, cause these chemicals to act as an agonist, partial agonist, or antagonist to a variety of endogenous hormones. Many organochlorine pesticides (including DDT, methoxychlor, and dicofol) have shown estrogen-like effects [11] or anti-androgen effects in animals [12]. Male children of mothers exposed to high doses of PCBs in Taiwan were found to have alterations of serum estradiol, serum testosterone, and follicle-stimulating hormone levels [13], as well as alterations in external genitalia [14]. In boys in the North Carolina PCB study, higher prenatal exposure to dicholorodiphenyldicholoroethylene (DDE), the DDT metabolite, was associated with greater height and weight at puberty [15]. Even as recently as 15 years ago, serum concentrations of DDE in humans were found at 100-fold greater levels than endogenous estradiol in premenopausal women and at about the same concentration as testosterone in men [16].

Thyroid hormone is essential for normal neurodevelopment of the fetus and young child. Various studies performed around the world have found alterations of thyroid hormones related to either in utero or childhood exposure to PCBs or dioxins [17,48,49]. Despite the variable effects of chemicals on thyroid-stimulating hormone, it seems that some of these compounds also may act on biologic systems that are not directly the result of thyroid hormone action (eg, through calcium signaling and increased reactive oxygen species) [18]. Additional studies in rats have demonstrated that PCBs can interfere with thyroid hormone signaling in the fetal brain by direct action on the fetus, absent changes in maternal thyroid status [19]. Recent studies have provided evidence that the effects of thyroid-disrupting chemicals are additive [20]. These findings in animal studies combined with the known influence of thyroid hormone on human neurocognitive development observed in epidemiologic studies have led to concerns about the effects of POPs on thyroid regulation and neurodevelopment in infants.

Two separate studies have demonstrated an association between DDE concentrations in maternal milk and shortened lactation time [50,51]. In developing nations longer duration of lactation is associated with increased infant survival. Although in some developing countries DDT has continued to be used in malaria control, a recent analysis suggests that the lives saved by DDT malaria control may be more than offset by infant deaths caused by reduced nutrition and increased diarrheal diseases attributable to the adverse effects of DDT on duration of lactation and increases in preterm birth [52].

Immune effects

Animal research has shown dioxin exposure to be associated with thymic atrophy, down-regulation of cytotoxic T- or B-lymphocyte differentiation, poorer antibody response, and reduced lymphocyte activation [21]. For the Taiwanese cohort exposed in utero, children were found to have a 25% decrease in IgA levels ($P < .01$), a 40% decrease in IgM levels ($P < .001$), and a 50% reduction in helper/suppressor T-cell ratio. A five- to six-fold increased risk of pneumonia/bronchitis and middle ear disease was reported in these children [22]. Similarly, a study of Inuit children revealed a significant association between elevated prenatal pesticide exposures to DDE and hexachlorobenzene and a higher incidence of otitis media in the first year of life (an approximately 50% increase) [23]. A significant negative association between serum dioxin levels and plasma IgG was still evident 20 years after exposure resulting from a large industrial accident in Seveso, Italy, with a nearly 25% difference in IgG levels between the highest and lowest exposed quartiles [24].

In the Dutch cohort described previously, prenatal PCB and dioxin exposure was found to be associated with changes in T lymphocytes [25]. A follow-up study in this group of children demonstrated that immune effects associated with prenatal PCB exposure (including higher number of lymphocytes and T-cell markers and lower mumps and measles antibodies) persist into childhood [26]. Further evidence for an alteration of immune function was seen in a study of Flemish children in whom there was a negative association between PCB levels and IgG, IgE, and allergic responses [27].

The mechanism for immunosuppression by POPs is poorly understood. Some hypotheses suggest that these molecules bind to the aryl hydrocarbon receptor and thereby alter the expression of genes involved in cell differentiation and proliferation of immune cells. In vitro studies also have suggested that dioxins and PCBs may alter thymus maturation and thymocyte differentiation [28].

Cancers

Many of the POPs are classified as possible or probable human carcinogens. Heptachlor epoxide, dieldrin, oxychlordane, and DDE have been associated with an 80% to 240% increase in risk of non-Hodgkin's lymphoma [29]. In the case of DDT, animal data suggest an increase in liver cancer, lung cancer, and lymphoma [30], and human studies report an association with non-Hodgkin's lymphoma (odds ratio, 4.5; 95% confidence interval, 1.7–12.0) [31]. Table 1 summarizes the cancer classifications in the California Safe Drinking Water and Toxic Enforcement Act of 1986, the most comprehensive authoritative list of carcinogens. PCBs have been classified as probable human carcinogens based on limited human data and significant animal data. In humans, studies of occupationally exposed electrical workers reveal an increased risk of malignant melanoma, biliary cancer, stomach cancer, and thyroid cancer. In the Taiwanese cohort exposed to PCB-contaminated rice oil, there was excess mortality from all types of malignancies, especially of the liver and lung [30].

Dioxin, specifically 2,3,7,8-TCDD, has the notoriety of being classified as a known human carcinogen based on both human and animal data. In animals, low-dose exposure to 2,3,7,8-TCDD and other dioxins causes cancer in several sites in multiple species. Four cohorts of occupationally exposed workers demonstrate that dioxins are a potent multisite carcinogen (including non-Hodgkin's lymphoma, soft tissue sarcoma, and respiratory cancers), similar to smoking and ionizing radiation [28].

Emerging persistent organic pollutants

The experiences from the mostly banned Stockholm POPs provide a framework for understanding the possible range of toxicities that POPs may have on human health. This experience also has emphasized the importance of prevention and global regulation. Several other emerging POPs have come to public attention. These newer POPs pose potential concerns, although they do not yet have strong epidemiologic data to support negative effects on human health. These concerns arise from their similarities, both structurally and functionally, to previous POPs combined with characteristic bioaccumulation, transplacental transfer, and transfer to breast milk. Although many human health risks are not yet proven, a precautionary approach can be helpful for minimizing human risk.

Polybrominated diphenyl ethers

(PBDEs) have been used for the past 30 years as flame retardants in plastics, wire insulation, electrical parts, printed circuit boards, polyurethane foam, and textiles (such as carpets and draperies). They are structurally similar to PCBs and seem to have a mode of action that also includes disruption of the thyroid hormone system [32]. Animal studies suggest the PBDEs, like PCBs, have effects on learning and behavior and that the neurobehavioral effects of PBDEs and PCBs may be additive [53]. In utero exposure to PBDEs in rats has resulted in delayed puberty and decreased ovarian follicles in females and in decreased circulating sex steroids and feminization of sexually dimorphic behavior in adult males [54]. At this time, there are only limited animal data and insufficient human data for carcinogenicity classification.

Like other POPs, the PBDEs resist degradation and are lipophilic, thus accumulating in fat. The half-lives of various congeners of PBDEs in humans vary from 1 week to 3 months. Until recently, an estimated 70,000 tons were produced each year, mostly as pentaBDE, octaBDE, and deca-BDE, (named for the number of bromine atoms). Although increasing levels have been detected in aquatic sediment, public health concern was raised when these chemicals were detected in the Swedish breast milk–monitoring program in 1998 [55]. Comparison with archived breast milk samples detected a logarithmic increase in concentrations over a 20-year period, as depicted in Fig. 2. There has been evidence of a decline in breast milk levels of PBDEs (Fig. 2) in Sweden since efforts began to eliminate use there.

Ensuing studies in animals, food, and humans revealed a similar pattern of rapidly increasing levels worldwide [30]. The levels of PBDEs are estimated to be 10 to 40 times higher in North American populations than in Europeans [56].

The major routes of exposure to PBDEs seem to be dietary intake and direct indoor exposure to PBDEs in air and dust. Some studies have indicated that meat and fish currently may be a less important source of exposure than for PCBs [57]. Although originally there was little concern about decaBDE, because it is not as readily absorbed after oral intake, recent studies suggest that decaBDE is biologically available and can accumulate in predator species [58]. In addition, decaBDE may degrade in the environment to lower brominated forms that are more easily absorbable and more toxicologically active [59]. Perhaps 5% of the United States population (15 million people) carry body burdens of PBDEs associated with alterations of reproductive organs in rats and within an order of magnitude of those causing neurodevelopmental effects in mice [60]. Current exposures to inhabitants of the United States leave little margin of safety.

Nitromusks

Synthetic musks are a component of many fragrances including soaps, cosmetics, and detergents. Most industrial musk production consists of two major classes of compounds, monocyclic nitroaromatic musks (nitromusks) and polycyclic musks. Musk xylene and musk ketone belong to the nitromusk category of compounds. Production is estimated to be 2000 tons per year. The high lipophilicity and propensity to bioconcentrate have led to comparisons with PCBs and other POPs. These chemicals have been detected in surface water and fish [61]. Further, the presence of these substances in human milk and adipose tissue has attracted concern [62]. Half-life in the human body has been estimated at approximately 3 months [63]. Current opinion favors the hypothesis that most nitromusk exposure occurs through dermal application of musk-containing products [64].

Comprehensive toxicologic studies on long-term effects are lacking for this class of compounds. Some animal studies have shown evidence for neurologic and hepatic toxicity [65]. There also is evidence of increased rates of benign and malignant liver tumors in mice [62]. Although there is no evidence for genotoxicity, some studies have suggested that musk ketone may act as a comutagen. Additionally, musk ketone has been shown to be a potent inducer of cytochrome P-450 enzymes; musk xylene can either inhibit or induce these enzymes [66].

Many countries have taken action to limit production of nitromusks. Japan has banned their use, German industry has voluntarily halted production, and the United States forbids their use in products that may be ingested but allows their use in products for dermal application. Preliminary evidence suggests that there has been a decrease in human serum levels in Germany since the discontinuation of production in 1993 [67].

Lindane

Lindane (gamma-hexachlorocyclohexane) has been used since the 1940s throughout the world as a pesticide on crops and animals and as treatment for human head lice and scabies. Because of concerns about this chemical's persistence and bioaccumulation, potential carcinogenicity, and effects on the endocrine systems of animals, it has been banned or severely restricted in at least 85 countries. In the United States most agricultural uses have been eliminated. Extensive use in many countries persists and has resulted in contamination of products significant to children, such as milk and butter [68]. In the United States and elsewhere, its poor safety profile and marginal efficacy has resulted in lindane being considered of limited pharmaceutical usefulness. Currently the Food and Drug Administration provides cautions about the use of lindane in persons weighing less than 110 pounds because of potential neurotoxicity [69].

In 2002 California banned the use of pharmaceutical lindane. The Los Angeles Sanitation District reported that one application for head lice could contaminate 6 million gallons of waste water above acceptable limits for aquatic ecosystems. A public draft report from the Commission on Environmental Cooperation suggests there have been no reports of significant difficulties resulting from the California ban [70].

Perfluorooctanesulfonate and perfluorooctanoic acid

Perfluorooctanoic acid (PFOA) and perfluorooctanesulfonate (PFOS) are perfluorinated compounds that are used as synthetic surfactants in lubricants, paints, cosmetics, and fire-fighting foam, on water-repellent clothing, in food packaging, and in nonstick pans. They are stable in the environment, and some studies have shown no evident biodegradation and a half-life of 96 years. In studies in occupationally exposed workers, biologic half-life has been estimated at 4.4 years. Further, these chemicals now have been detected in blood sera of the general pediatric population [71]. In a study of blood concentrations of various chemicals around the world, the United States and Poland were found to have the highest levels of PFOS [72].

In animals, studies have shown decreased hematocrit and thyroid hormones associated with PFOA. PFOA seems to interfere with fatty acid metabolism and cholesterol synthesis [73]. Cancer bioassays have shown an increase in testicular, liver, and mammary tumors from PFOA exposure. At high doses in monkeys, PFOS has been associated with lower triiodothyronine and estradiol levels and with increased liver weight [74]. PFOS at high doses also has been associated consistently with lowered cholesterol and metabolic wasting in animals [75]. In contrast, human epidemiologic data have shown a positive association between PFOA levels and cholesterol, triglycerides, and triiodothyronine [76]. In studies of PFOS, there has been possible association with bladder cancer [77], malignant melanoma, and colonic tumors [78].

At this point, it is unclear whether current levels could be harmful to humans. The persistence and prolonged half-life of these substances may cause a gradual increase in background levels, however. Although in 2000 the largest producer of PFOA compounds voluntarily announced the intention to stop producing these chemicals, a different major chemical company quickly began producing them. In 2006 the US Environmental Protection Agency (EPA) announced the voluntary PFOA Stewardship Program that aims to elicit corporate commitments to reduce emissions and use of these chemicals by 95% by 2010 globally. At this time, it is unclear what exposures carry the highest risk. Some data have suggested that drinking water [79] and residential area [80] may play the largest role. Other research has pointed out that perfluorochemicals are used in small quantities in substances that come into contact with food, such as nonstick cookware coatings (PFOA) and paper coatings for moisture resistance (eg, microwave popcorn bags, pizza boxes, PFOS) [81]. The extent to which these chemicals are transferred to food and the impact of heat on this process is not yet clear.

Anticipatory guidance

In the United States, research has shown a significant decline in the body burden of dioxins and PCBs from 1972 to 1999; however, this decrease seems to have leveled off from 1999 to 2003 [82]. The decreases probably are attributable to bans on many of these substances. Exposure to most POPs occurs gradually over time without any overt symptoms. Because these substances are pervasive in the environment, highly persistent within the body, and lack any viable elimination options, the most important factor in minimizing adverse health effects is reduction of exposure. Although reducing exposure ideally involves removal of these chemicals from commerce, or regulation of their use, there is some role for measures to reduce individual exposure. Counseling patients, especially young women before childbearing age, on avoidance of potentially high sources of POPs exposures and allaying unnecessary fears about breastfeeding can promote good health habits across generations.

Diet

The EPA estimates that 90% of dioxin exposure occurs from diet. Foods that contain the highest concentrations of POPs include high-fat cuts of beef, bacon, frankfurters, full-fat cheeses, butter, and fatty fish (eg, farm-raised salmon) [83]. Within these same categories are foods with lower concentrations of these contaminants, including shrimp, lean ham, lean steak, cottage cheese, and margarine [36]. Other recommendations include using vegetable oils instead of animal fats, trimming the excess skin and fat from meat, and choosing lean cuts of meat. Also, washing vegetables and peeling root and waxy-coated vegetables is recommended [84]. Changing a mother's diet during pregnancy or lactation will not significantly reduce the levels of most POPs and resulting exposures to the fetus or infant, because the mother's contribution reflects her long-term exposure. Rather, efforts to counsel and educate individuals about a diet low in animal fats should begin in childhood, so that women enter their reproductive years with a minimal body burden of potentially fetotoxic substances.

Researchers have demonstrated an association between increasing half-life of dioxins and increasing age and adiposity. This finding suggests that the youngest children may be able to excrete these substances more readily. By adolescence, however, the stability of these substances within the body becomes prolonged. For this reason, institution of a diet that is relatively low in animal fat at a young age is helpful. Fatty fish, although a source of important nutrients, is also a significant source of POPs exposure. Therefore, cooking fish in a manner that allows juices to drain away and moderate consumption (one or two meals per week) of a variety of fish types is suggested.

Breastfeeding

Much public concern has arisen regarding the concentrations of POPs in breast milk and the effects on the neonate. Overall, the epidemiologic research has demonstrated the strongest adverse effects on cognitive function to be associated with prenatal concentrations of PCBs and dioxins in cord blood, rather than with concentrations in breast milk. Presently, there is no recommendation to reduce breastfeeding. In fact, the American Academy of Pediatrics recommends exclusive breastfeeding until the age of 6 months [38]. The benefits of breastfeeding to the infant, mother, and society are clear and positive and outweigh the potential risks posed by pollutant exposure. Although infant formula does not contain significant amounts of POPs, studies comparing formula-fed and breastfed infants consistently show that breastfed babies are healthier and have better neurologic functioning [85]. Additionally, it has been demonstrated that prolonged breastfeeding leads to progressively lower levels of PCBs and dioxins in breast milk; therefore, there does not seem to be a benefit to shortening the duration of breastfeeding [86].

Although breastfeeding is the general recommendation for the public, some subgroups may warrant further consideration. Women with occupational exposures to POPs or other related chemicals (eg, waste-incineration workers, cosmetics industry workers, electronics workers, farm workers) or people involved in a disaster incident may require biomonitoring and risk–benefit evaluation. Additionally, families who fish for subsistence or ethnic groups that consume large quantities of seafood may require more careful assessment. In unusual circumstances, the advice of state health department officials may be sought for specific regions in which high concentrations may be present in the environment.

Consumer products

In addition to dietary counseling, anticipatory guidance may include education about consumer products. Theoretically, bleached paper products (eg, coffee filters, tampons, diapers) may contain small amounts of dioxin. The reaction between chlorine and lignins in wood fiber can result in the formation of many chlorinated organic compounds including dioxin. The amounts are very small, however, especially compared with the magnitude of dietary exposures. Concerned consumers generally can find unbleached or chlorine-free paper products if they choose.

PBDEs may be present as an additive flame retardant in polyurethane-foam mattresses, cushions, and pillows as well as in draperies and carpet padding. Unlike reactive flame retardants, additive flame retardants are more likely to leach and volatilize into the environment. Additionally, there is a risk of PBDE volatilization from the plastic casing of computers, television sets, and other electronic devices. There are very few data on the magnitude of exposure to PBDE from these sources. The type of PBDE used as a flame retardant in polyurethane foam has been banned recently in several states and in the European Union. The EPA has come to a voluntary agreement with the major manufacturer of this product to phaseout production, so it is likely that newer mattresses, cushions, and pillows will be free of these chemicals. Many major corporations now report on their Web sites that they manufacture PBDE-free computers, televisions, monitors, electrical equipment, and mattresses.

Recent concern over the potential release of PFOS/PFOA from nonstick cookware and from food packaging has caused some alarm [75]. The health effects of low-level exposure from food cooked or stored in contact with these substances or from inhalation of material off-gassing during cooking are uncertain. PFOS also is used as a rain repellent in clothing, as a carpet spot cleaner, in fire-fighting foams, and as an artificial wax for some sporting equipment such as skis and snowboards. Because there is no centralized list of products that contain PFOS/PFOA, and because the exposures from existing sources have not been quantified, it remains difficult for physicians to give useful anticipatory guidance to patients at this time.

Nitromusk exposure can occur from a variety of consumer products in the United States. Although the use of nitromusks has been banned for products that may be ingested, they are still present in many cosmetics including laundry detergents, perfumes, air fresheners, hand creams, and soaps. Because these chemicals seem to penetrate the skin, dermal exposure is a concern. The precautionary principle suggests that it may be prudent to minimize the use of nitromusk-containing cosmetics in children and women of childbearing age. Unfortunately, nitromusk compounds are not specifically identified on product labels, which instead simply indicate the presence of "fragrance." Products that are unscented or that contain only natural fragrances are not likely to contain nitromusks.

The issue of POPs in consumer products affects individual patients and also the environment as a whole. These products can cause environmental contamination and possible health effects in future generations if the chemicals persist and bioaccumulate after disposal. Although there currently is no program for appropriate disposal of many products that contain newer POPs, some states have begun to collect electronic waste for recycling and proper disposal.

Laboratory testing

Laboratory testing for the presence of POPs in blood or breast milk in the general population is not generally recommended. Testing can be expensive and difficult to interpret. Most laboratories do not have standard procedures for these tests, and government laboratories may be required. For many POPs, laboratories do not have an established reference range, especially for media such as breast milk. In the setting of occupational exposures to chemicals, an occupational physician can arrange biomonitoring for specific chemicals or their metabolites. Overall, routine laboratory testing carries high expense and poor reliability and therefore is not a good screening method. The best method for reducing exposure to most POPs is prevention through timely patient education.

Summary

Diagnosis of elevated exposures to POPs can be difficult, and treatment options are limited or nonexistent. The optimal method for prevention involves international elimination of these chemicals. Efforts to counsel and educate individuals should begin in their childhood, so that good eating habits are established and women enter their reproductive years with a minimal body burden of potentially fetotoxic substances. Breast milk remains the healthiest and safest form of nutrition for newborn babies. Despite increasing regulatory efforts to curtail production of most POPs, they will continue to persist in the environment, ecosystem, and food supply for years to come.

Acknowledgments

The authors thank Carianne Galik Miller for her editorial assistance and Gail DeRita for assistance with the endnotes and formatting.

References

[1] Schafer KS, Kegley SE. Persistent toxic chemicals in the US food supply. J Epidemiol Community Health 2002;56:813–7.

[2] Stockholm Convention on Persistent Organic Pollutants. Available at: http://www.pops.int/. Accessed March 27, 2006.

[3] Vreugdenhil HJ, Lanting CI, Mulder PG, et al. Effects of prenatal PCB and dioxin background exposure on cognitive and motor abilities in Dutch children at school age. J Pediatr 2002;140(1):48–56.

[4] Fein GG, Jacobson JL, Joacobson SW, et al. Prenatal exposure to polychlorinated biphenyls: effects on birth size and gestational age. J Pediatr 1984;105(2):315–9.

[5] Lonky E, Reihman J, Darvill T, et al. Neonatal behavioral assessment scale performance in humans influenced by maternal consumption of environmentally contaminated Lake Orntario fish. J Great Lakes Res 1996;22(2):198–212.

[6] Darvill T, Lonky E, Reihman J. Prenatal exposure to PCBs and infant performance on the Fagan test of infant intelligence. Neurotoxicology 2000;21:1029–38.

[7] Jacobson JL, Jacobon SW, Humphrey HEB. Effects of *in utero* exposure to polychlorinated biphenyls and related contaminants on cognitive functioning in young children. J Pediatr 1990;116:38–45.

[8] Jacobson JL, Jacobson SW. Intellectual impairment in children exposed to polychlorinated biphenyls *in utero*. N Engl J Med 1996;335(11):783–9.

[9] Rogan WJ. Neonatal effects of transplacental exposure to PCBs and DDE. J Pediatr 1986;109:335–41.

[10] Gladen BC, Rogan WJ. Effects of perinatal polychlorinated biphenyls and dichlorodiphenyl dichloroethane on later development. J Pediatr 1991;119:58–63.

[11] Guillette LJ Jr, Brock JW, Rooney AA, et al. Serum concentrations of various environmental contaminants and their relationship to sex steroid concentrations and phallus size in juvenile American alligators. Arch Environ Contam Toxicol 1999;36(4):447–55.

[12] Kelce WR, Stone CR, Laws SC, et al. Persistent DDT metabolite p,p'-DDE is a potent androgen receptor antagonist. Nature 1995;375(6532):581–5.

[13] Hsu PC, Lai TJ, Guo NW, et al. Serum hormones in boys prenatally exposed to polychlorinated biphenyls and dibenzofurans. J Toxicol Environ Health 2005;68(17–18):1447–56.

[14] Guo YL, Lai TJ, Ju SH. Sexual development and biological findings in Yucheng children. Chemosphere 1993;14:235–8.

[15] Rogan WJ, Ragan NB. Evidence of effects of environmental chemicals on the endocrine system in children. Pediatrics 2003;112:247–52.

[16] Stehr-Green PA. Demographic and seasonal influences on human serum pesticide residue levels. J Toxicol Environ Health 1989;27:405–21.

[17] Osius N, Karmaus W, Kruse H. Exposure to polychlorinated biphenyls and levels of thyroid hormones in children. Environ Health Perspect 1999;107(10):843–9.

[18] Sharlin DS, Bansal R, Zoeller RT. Polychlorinated biphenyls exert selective effects on cellular composition of white matter in a manner inconsistent with thyroid hormone insufficiency. Endocrinology 2006;147(2):846–58.

[19] Gauger KJ, Kato Y, Haraguchi K, et al. Polychlorinated biphenyls (PCBs) exert thyroid hormone-like effects in the fetal rat brain but do not bind to thyroid hormone receptors. Environ Health Perspect 2004;112(5):516–23.

[20] Crofton KM, Craft ES, Hedge JM, et al. Thyroid-hormone-disrupting chemicals: evidence for dose dependent additivity or synergism. Environ Health Perspect 2005;113:1549–54.

[21] Kim HA, Kim EM, Park YC, et al. Immunotoxicological effects of Agent Orange exposure to the Vietnam War Korean veterans. Ind Health 2003;41(3):158–66.

[22] Rogan WJ, Gladd BC, Hung KL, et al. Congenital poisoning by polychlorinated biphenyls and their contaminants in Taiwan. Science 1988;241:334–6.

[23] Dewailly E, Ayotte P, Bruneau S, et al. Susceptibility to infections and immune status in Inuit infants exposed to organochlorines. Environ Health Perspect 2000;108(3):205–10.

[24] Baccarelli A, Mocarelli P, Patterson DG, et al. Immunologic effects of dioxin: new results from Seveso and comparison with other studies. Environ Health Perspect 2002;110(12): 1169–73.

[25] Weisglas-Kuperus N, Sas TC, Koopman-Esseboom C, et al. Immunologic effects of background prenatal and postnatal exposure to dioxins and polychlorinated biphenyls in Dutch infants. Pediatr Res 1995;38(3):404–10.

[26] Weisglas-Kuperus N, Patandin S, Berbers GAM, et al. Immunologic effects of background exposure to polychlorinated biphenyls and dioxins in Dutch preschool children. Environ Health Perspect 2000;108(12):1203–7.

[27] Van Den Heuvel RL, Koppen G, Staessen JA, et al. Immunologic biomarkers in relation to exposure markers of PCBs and dioxins in Flemish adolescents (Belgium). Environ Health Perspect 2002;110(6):595–600.

[28] Lai ZW, Fiore NC, Gasiewitcz TA, et al. 2,3,7,8-tetrachlorodibenzo-p-dioxin and diethylstilbestrol affect thymocytes at different stages of development in fetal thymus organ culture. Toxicol Appl Pharmacol 1998;149:167–77.

[29] Quintana PJ, Delfino RJ, Korrick S, et al. Adipose tissue levels of organochlorine pesticides and polychlorinated biphenyls and risk of non-Hodgkin's lymphoma. Environ Health Perspect 2004;112(8):854–61.

[30] International Agency for Research on Cancer. Overall evaluations of carcinogenicity: an updating of IARC monographs volumes 1-42. Supplement 7. Lyon (France): World Health Organization; 1987. p. 322–6.

[31] Rothman N, Cantor KP, Blair A, et al. A nested case-control study of non-Hodgkin lymphoma and serum organochlorine residues. Lancet 1997;350:240–4.

[32] McDonald TA. A perspective on the potential health risks of PBDEs. Chemosphere 2002; 46(5):745–55.

[33] Fisher BE. Most unwanted: persistent organic pollutants. Environ Health Perspect 1999; 107(1):A18–23.

[34] Brunstrom B, Halldin K. Ecotoxicological risk assessment of environmental pollutants in the Arctic. Toxicol Lett 2000;15(112):111–8.

[35] Solomon GM, Weiss P. Chemical contaminants in breast milk: time trends and regional variability. Environ Health Perspect 2002;110(6):A339–47.

[36] Committee on the Implications of Dioxin in the Food Supply. Dioxins and dioxin-like compounds in the food supply: strategies to decrease exposure. Washington, DC: National Academies Press; 2003. p. 116–120.

[37] Patandin S, Dagnelie PC, Mulder PG, et al. Dietary exposure to polychlorinated biphenyls and dioxins from infancy until adulthood: a comparison between breast-feeding, toddler, and long-term exposure. Environ Health Perspect 1999;107(1):45–51.

[38] Gartner LM, Morton J, Lawrence RA, et al. American Academy of Pediatrics Section on Breastfeeding. Policy statement: breastfeeding and the use of human milk. Pediatrics 2005; 115(2):496–506.

[39] Brouwer A, Ahlborg UG, van Leeuwen FX, et al. Report of the WHO working group on the assessment of the health risks for human infants from exposure to PCDDs, PCDFs, and PCBs. Chemosphere 1998;37(9–12):1627–43.

[40] Longnecker MP, Rogan WJ, Lucier G. The Human health effects of DDT and PCBs and an overview of organochlorines in public health. Annu Rev Public Health 1997;18:211–44.

[41] Pirkle JL, Wolfe WH, Patterson DG, et al. Estimates of the half-life of 2,3,7,8-tetrachlorodibenzo-p-dioxin in Vietnam veterans of operation ranch hand. J Toxicol Environ Health 1989;27(2):165–71.

[42] Nguon K, Baxter MG, Sajdel-Sulkowska EM, et al. Perinatal exposure to polychlorinated biphenyls differentially affects cerebellar development and motor functions in male and female rat neonates. Cerebellum 2005;4(2):112–22.

[43] Chen YC, Guo YL, Hsu CC, et al. Cognitive development of Yu-Cheng ("oil disease") children prenatally exposed to heat-degraded PCBs. JAMA 1992;268(22):3213–8.

[44] Patandin S, Koopman-Esseboom C, de Riddr MA, et al. Effects of environmental exposure to polychlorinated biphenyls and dioxins on birth size and growth in Dutch children. Pedeatr Res 1998;44(4):538–45.

[45] Koopman-Esseboom C, Weisglas-Kuperus N, de Ridder MA, et al. Effects of polychlorinated biphenyl/dioxin exposure and feeding type on infants' mental and psychomotor development. Pediatrics 1996;97(5):700–6.

[46] Porterfield S. Vulnerability of the developing brain to thyroid abnormalities: environmental insults to the thyroid system. Environ Health Perspect 1994;102:125–30.

[47] Eskenazi B, Marks AR, Bradman A, et al. In Utero exposure to dichlorodiphenyltrichloroethane (DDT) and dichlorodiphenyldichloroethylene (DDE) and neurodevelopment among young Mexican American children. Pediatrics 2006;118:233–41.

[48] Pluim HJ, de Vijlder JJ, Olie K. Effects of pre- and postnatal exposure to chlorinated dioxins and furans on human neonatal thyroid hormone concentrations. Environ Health Perspect 1993;101(6):504–8.

[49] Koopman-Esseboom C, Morse DC, Weisglas-Kuperus N, et al. Effects of dioxins and polychlorinated biphenyls on thyroid hormone status of pregnant women and their infants. Pediatr Res 1994;36(4):468–73.

[50] Rogan WJ, Gladen BC, McKinney JD, et al. Polychlorinated biphenyls and dichlorodiphenyl dichloroethylene in human milk: effects on growth, morbidity and duration of lactation. Am J Public Health 1987;77:1294–7.

[51] Gladen BC, Rogan WJ. DDE and shortened duration of lactation in a Northern Mexican town. Am J Public Health 1995;85:504–8.

[52] Rogan WJ, Chen A. Health risks and benefits of bis (4-chlorophenyl)-1,1,1-trichloroethane (DDT). Lancet 2005;366(9487):763–73.

[53] Eriksson P, Fischer C, Fredriksson A. Co-exposure to a polybrominated diphenyl ether (PBDE 99) and an ortho-substituted PCB (PCB 52) enhances developmental neurotoxic effects. Organohalogen Compounds 2003;61:81–3.

[54] Lilienthal H, Hack A, Roth-Harer A, et al. Effects of developmental exposure to 2,2,4,4,5-pentabromodiphenyl ether (PBDE-99) on sex steroids, sexual development, and sexually dimorphic behavior in rats. Environ Health Perspect 2006;114(2):194–201.

[55] Hooper K, She J. Lessons from the PBDEs: precautionary principle, primary prevention, and the value of community based body burden monitoring using breast milk. Environ Health Perspect 2003;111(1):109–14.

[56] Schecter A, Papke O, Tung KC, et al. Polybrominated diphenyl ether flame retardants in the U.S. population: current levels, temporal trends, and comparison with dioxins, dibenzofurans, and polychlorinated biphenyls. J Occup Environ Med 2005;47(3):199–211.

[57] Morland KB, Landrigan PJ, Sjodin A, et al. Body burdens of polybrominated diphenyl ethers among urban anglers. Environ Health Perspect 2005;113(12):1689–92.

[58] Lindberg P, Sellstrom U, Haggberg L, et al. Higher brominated diphenyl ethers and hexabromocyclododecane found in eggs of peregrine falcons (Falco peregrinus) breeding in Sweden. Environ Sci Technol 2004;38(1):93–6.

[59] Eriksson J, Green N, Marsh G, et al. Photochemical decomposition of 15 polybrominated diphenyl ether congeners in methanol/water. Environ Sci Technol 2004;38(11):3119–25.

[60] McDonald TA. Polybrominated diphenylether levels among United States residents: daily intake and risk of harm to the developing brain and reproductive organs. Integrated Environmental Assessment and Management 2005;1(4):343–54.

[61] Rimkus G, Wof M. Nitro musk fragrances in biota from freshwater and marine environments. Chemosphere 1995;30:641–51.

[62] Liebl B, Ehrenstorfer S. Nitromusks in human milk. Chemosphere 1993;27:2253–60.

[63] Liebl B, Mayer R, Ommer S, et al. Transition of nitro musks and polycyclic musks into human milk. Adv Exp Med Biol 2000;478:289–305.

[64] Hawkins DR, Ford RA. Dermal absorption and disposition of musk ambrette, musk ketone and musk xylene in rats. Toxicol Lett 1999;111(1–2):95–103.

[65] Maekawa A, Matsushima Y, Onodera H, et al. Long-term toxicity/carcinogenicity of musk xylol in B6C3F1 mice. Food Chem Toxicol 1990;28:581–6.

[66] Stuard SB, Caudill D, Lehman-McKeeman LD. Characterization of effects of musk ketone on mouse hepatic cytochrome P450 enzymes. Fundam Appl Toxicol 1997;40: 264–71.

[67] Kafferlein HE, Angerer J. Trends in the musk xylene concentrations in plasma samples from the general population from 1992/1993 to 1998 and the relevance of dermal uptake. Int Arch Occup Environ Health 2001;74:470–6.

[68] Waliszewski SM, Villalobos-Pietrini R, Gomez-Arroyo S, et al. Persistent organochlorine pesticide levels in cow's milk samples from tropical regions of Mexico. Food Addit Contam 2003;20(3):270–5.

[69] FDA package labeling. Available at: http://www.fda.gov/cder/foi/label/2003/006309sham poolbl.pdf. Accessed March 12, 2006.

[70] CEC 2006. The North American Regional Action Plan (NARAP) on lindane and other hex-achlorocyclohexane (HCH) isomers. Montreal (Canada): Commission for Environmental Cooperation. Available at: http://www.cec.org/pubs_docs/documents/index.cfm?varlan=english&ID=2053. Accessed January 9, 2007.

[71] Olsen GW, Burris JM, Lundberg JK, et al. Identification of fluorochemicals in human sera. III. Pediatric participants in a group A Streptococci clinical trial investigation; 2002. Final Report, 3M Medical Department. Available at: http://www.chemicalindustryarchives.org/. Accessed March 29, 2006.

[72] Kannan K, Corsolini S, Falandysz J, et al. Perfluorooctanesulfonate and related fluorochem-icals in human blood from several countries. Environmental Science and Technology 2004; 38(17):4489–95.

[73] Haughom B, Spydevold O. The mechanism underlying the hypolipemic effect of perfluor-ooctanoic acid (PFOA), perfluorooctane sulphonic acid (PFOSA) and clofibric acid. Biochim Biophys Acta 1992;1128:65–72.

[74] Seacat AM, Thomford PJ, Hansen KJ, et al. Subchronic toxicity studies on perfluoroocta-nesulfonate potassium salt in Cynomolgus monkeys. Toxicol Sci 2002;68(1):249–64.

[75] Olsen GW, Burris JM, et al. Serum perfluorooctane sulfonate and hepatic and lipid clinical chemistry tests in fluorochemical production employees. J Occup Environ Med 1999;41(9): 799–806.

[76] Olsen GW, Burlew MM, Burris JM, et al. A cross-sectional analysis of serum perfluoroocta-nesulfonate (PFOS) and perfluorooctanoate (PFOA) in relation to clinical chemistry, thyroid hormone, hematology and urinalysis results from male and female employee participants of the 2000 Antwerp and Decatur fluorochemical medical surveillance program; 2001. Final Report, 3M Medical Department. Available at: http://www.chemicalindustryarchives.org/. Accessed March 29, 2006.

[77] Alexander BH, Olsen GW, Burris JM, et al. Mortality study of workers employed at a per-fluorooctanesulfonyl fluoride manufacturing facility. Occup Environ Med 2003;60:792–9.

[78] Olsen GW, Burlew MM, Marshall JC, et al. Analysis of episodes of care in a perfluoroocta-nesulfonyl fluoride production facility. J Occup Environ Med 2004;46(8):837–46.

[79] Norimitsu S, Harada K, Inoue K, et al. Perfluorooctanoate and perfluorooctane sulfonate concentrations in surface water in Japan. J Occup Health 2004;46:49–59.

[80] Harada K, Saito N, Inoue K, et al. The influence of time, sex and geographic factors on levels of perfluorooctane sulfonate and perfluorooctanoate in human serum over the last 25 years. J Occup Health 2004;46(2):141–7.

[81] Begley TH, White K, Honigfort P, et al. Perfluorochemicals: potential sources of and migra-tion from food packaging. Food Addit Contam 2005;22(10):1023–31.

[82] Hays SM, Aylward LL. Dioxin risks in perspective: past, present, and future. Regul Toxicol Pharmacol 2003;37(2):202–17.

[83] Hites RA, Foran JA, Schwager SJ, et al. Global assessment of polybrominated diphenyl ethers in farmed and wild salmon. Environ Sci Technol 2004;38:4945–59.

[84] Douglass JS, Murphy MM. Estimated exposure to dioxins in the food supply. Institute of medicine; Washington, DC: 2002.

[85] Leung AK, Sauve RS. Breast is best for babies. J Natl Med Assoc 2005;97(7):1010–9.

[86] Schecter A, Papke O, Lis A, et al. Decrease in milk and blood dioxin levels over two years in a mother nursing twins: estimates of decreased maternal and increased infant dioxin body burden from nursing. Chemosphere 1996;32(3):543–9.

PEDIATRIC CLINICS

OF NORTH AMERICA

Pediatr Clin N Am
54 (2007) 103–120

Indoor Environmental Influences on Children's Asthma

Hemant P. Sharma, MD[a],
Nadia N. Hansel, MD, MPH[b],
Elizabeth Matsui, MD, MHS[a],*,
Gregory B. Diette, MD, MHS[b],
Peyton Eggleston, MD[a], Patrick Breysse, PhD[c]

[a]*Division of Allergy and Immunology, Department of Pediatrics, Johns Hopkins University School of Medicine, 600 North Wolfe Street, CMSC 1102, Baltimore, MD 21287, USA*
[b]*Division of Pulmonary and Critical Care Medicine, Department of Medicine, Johns Hopkins University School of Medicine, 1830 East Monument Street, 5th floor, Baltimore, MD 21205, USA*
[c]*Department of Environmental Health Sciences, Johns Hopkins Bloomberg School of Public Health, 615 North Wolfe Street, E6630, Baltimore, MD 21205, USA*

The burden of asthma for children in the United States is substantial and has continued to rise for the past 2 decades [1–4]. Asthma generally is viewed as an illness that can be caused by and worsened by environmental factors, particularly among people who are genetically susceptible. The causes of the recent rise in asthma prevalence and morbidity remain largely speculative, but the relatively brief timescale of the change is most consistent with a change in environmental exposures, because a change in the genetic make-up would be expected to occur over generations rather than decades. Although much attention has been given to the outdoor environment, there is strong evidence that indoor exposure to allergens and pollutants has an important role in the pathogenesis of asthma. The indoor environment is particularly relevant, because most children spend the majority of time indoors, and the quality of the indoor environment is directly related to housing quality and lifestyle choices. This article reviews many of the indoor environmental factors for which there is evidence of a link to childhood asthma.

---

* Corresponding author.
E-mail address: ematsui@jhmi.edu (E. Matsui).

0031-3955/07/$ - see front matter © 2007 Elsevier Inc. All rights reserved.
doi:10.1016/j.pcl.2006.11.007
pediatric.theclinics.com

Allergen exposure and asthma

Allergens, and the immune response to them, have been implicated in asthma and the severity of the illness. Between 60% and 80% of children and young adults who have asthma have one or more positive skin tests to an aeroallergen, and those who are skin test–positive tend to have more severe asthma [5,6]. This finding suggests that exposure to certain allergens may contribute to disease severity. Furthermore, among inner-city asthmatics, where the burden of asthma is greatest in the United States, sensitivity to indoor allergens is more prevalent than sensitivity to outdoor allergens [7]. This article summarizes the findings of the effects of indoor allergens (dust mite, cockroach, cat and dog, and rodent) on asthma morbidity. It discusses the characteristics and epidemiology of each allergen, the relationship between exposure and sensitization, the effects on asthma, and the efficacy of avoidance or control measures.

Dust mite

House dust mite allergen was first identified in 1967 [8]. The major dust mite allergens, Der p 1 and Der p 2, are carried on relatively large particles (10–30 μm) that remain airborne only briefly [9]. The mites infest fabrics and are not particularly mobile. Disturbance is required for their allergen to be detected in the air. The distribution of house dust mite allergens varies widely in different homes [10,11], with highest concentrations found in the bedroom, especially in the bed. Mites require moisture; therefore, higher allergen levels are associated with increased moisture, such as in damp houses and basement bedrooms [12]. Allergen levels are also higher in summer than in winter [12].

There is evidence of a relationship between mite allergen exposure and skin test sensitization. Sensitization rates are much higher in communities with high mite concentrations [5]. In addition, the risk of sensitization increases linearly at concentrations higher than 2 μg/g of mite group 2 allergen [13]. A study of more than 1000 children in eight North American cities also found that exposure to high mite levels (> 10 ug/g) is associated with ninefold greater odds of skin test sensitization [14].

Based on all studies to date, the 2000 Institute of Medicine Report concluded there are causal relationships (1) between exposure to dust mite allergen and the development of asthma in susceptible children and (2) between exposure and asthma exacerbations in sensitized individuals [15]. The evidence cited includes studies in various countries demonstrating an association between dust mite sensitization and asthma (with odds ratios ≥ 6) [16], bronchial provocation experiments showing allergic response [17], and studies of clinical outcomes after mite allergen avoidance [18–25].

There is evidence that measures to control dust mite allergen are a reasonable approach to improving asthma in children, although whether the practices should be recommended on a larger scale remains controversial. The most effective method of control is the use of allergen-proof encasings fitted to the mattress and pillow [18,19]. Of more than a dozen clinical trials of allergen-proof encasings, seven have demonstrated a reduction in mite allergen and a clinical effect [19–25]. Dust mite covers are available by mail or in retail stores, are breathable and comfortable, and exclude nearly 100% of particles carrying mite allergen [26]. Although prior studies have found that allergen-proof bed covers can reduce mite allergen levels and improve clinical outcomes in selected populations, one recent study of more than 1100 adults suggests that providing encasings to all patients who have asthma may not be an effective public health intervention [27]. Washing sheets, pillowcases, blankets, and mattress pads at least weekly in warm water with detergent and with 8- to 10-minute cycles removes virtually all mite allergen [28]. Dry cleaning [29] and prolonged tumble-drying [30] effectively kill mites but are less effective at removing allergens. Vacuum cleaning reduces the bulk of household dust and reduces the overall exposure burden but does not change the concentration of mite allergen in settled dust [31]. Second-line measures for which there is evidence of mite allergen reduction include removal of wall-to-wall carpeting [32] and steam cleaning [26]. Other measures, which lack supporting evidence, include relocation of the bedroom [33] and application of acaracides [34]. The evidence surrounding dehumidifiers is inconsistent, with some studies showing a reduction in mite allergen levels [35], and others not [36].

Cockroach

Many cockroach allergens have been identified, but Bla g 1 and Bla g 2 are the most commonly tested in clinical studies. The sources of cockroach allergens may include saliva, fecal material, and secretions. Cockroach allergen particles, like dust mite allergens, are larger than 10 μm and are detectable in the air mainly after vigorous disturbance, with subsequent rapid settling [37]. Because cockroaches are highly mobile, allergen is widely distributed throughout a home and is highly concentrated in cracks and crevices. The highest levels of allergen typically are found in the kitchen, with somewhat lower levels in dust samples from sofas, bedding, and bedroom floors [38]. Of note, approximately 20% to 48% of homes without visible cockroaches still contain detectable cockroach allergen in dust samples [39,40].

Multiple studies have established the link between cockroach exposure and allergic sensitization. Cockroach allergen and sensitization occurs in both urban and rural areas, and detectable home exposure to cockroach is associated with an increase in the odds of a positive skin test response [14]. In addition, there is a dose–response relationship between cockroach allergen exposure and sensitization in asthmatic children [39,41]. Specifically, the National Cooperative Inner City Asthma Study (NCICAS) study showed that the risk of sensitization increases at very low exposures and that levels above 4 units of allergen per gram of settled dust do not seem to be associated with a substantial increase in risk [39].

The 2000 Institute of Medicine Report found sufficient evidence for a causal relationship between cockroach allergen exposure and exacerbation of asthma in sensitized individuals [15]. This conclusion was based on several findings, including an increase in asthma-related health care use in cockroach-exposed and -sensitized inner-city children [42]. The report also concluded that there is limited evidence from prospective birth cohort studies of an association between cockroach allergen exposure and the development of asthma in infants and young children [43], but that evidence is insufficient to support a similar association in older children [15].

The primary method of cockroach control is insecticide treatment aimed at reducing the allergen source [44]. A number of effective pesticides are available in gels or baits that are capable of reducing cockroach populations within 2 to 4 weeks, with sustained reductions for at least 3 months [45–47]. Reductions in cockroach populations are even longer if families change cleaning practices to remove sources that will attract reinfestation. Although no intervention studies have evaluated resultant pesticide levels in exposed children, it would be prudent to use traps, gels, and baits rather than sprays and dusts to minimize exposure of children to pesticides. Some trials of insecticide application have shown that cockroach populations can be reduced by more than 90% [44], whereas allergen levels may decline more slowly over 6 months. For example, one study showed that insecticide application with careful bait placement, guided by inspection, may be associated with a large reduction in cockroach allergen [48]. The degree of allergen reduction is sometimes found to be trivial, however [49,50], and, in heavily contaminated areas, treated rooms may still contain allergen at levels that have been associated with disease. Furthermore, in NCICAS phase 2, the intervention (education, professional pest control, cleaning) was successful in reducing asthma morbidity [51], but neither the cockroach numbers nor the level of cockroach allergen was reduced [49]. Therefore, there is conflicting evidence regarding the relationship between cockroach-control interventions and allergen reduction, and there is inadequate evidence relating to improvement of disease with interventions.

Cat and dog

Cat and dog allergens, unlike dust mite and cockroach allergens, are carried on small particles that remain airborne and are very adherent to surfaces and clothing [52]. These properties lead to widespread distribution, so that cat and dog allergen can be detected even in public buildings such as schools [53,54]. Allergen is brought to school on the clothing of children who have pets at home, and the highest airborne allergen levels occur around the desks of those children [53]. Cat and dog allergen, obviously, is found in homes with these pets; the allergens also can be found in homes without a pet, although the concentrations are 10 to 1000 times lower than in homes with a pet [55,56].

Study findings regarding the relationship between cat and dog exposure and specific sensitization are inconsistent [57]. Some studies show cat owners to be at increased risk of allergic sensitization [58], but other studies show a decreased risk [14,59]. Results are more consistent for dogs, suggesting that dog exposure has no effect or indeed may be protective against the development of specific sensitization to dog allergen [14,58]. In addition, persons without direct pet exposure in the home often show evidence of sensitization, possibly caused by the ubiquitous distribution of cat and dog allergens [57].

For both cat and dog, there is considerable evidence supporting a relationship between allergen exposure and exacerbation of asthma in sensitized individuals [15]. Studies of environmental allergen challenges (in "cat rooms") and bronchial allergen challenges show that cat-sensitized asthmatics develop asthma symptoms and decreased lung function in response to airborne cat allergen, even at low levels [55,60,61]. There are no analogous "dog room" studies; however, bronchial provocation with dog allergen does lead to decreased pulmonary function in dog-sensitized asthmatics [62,63]. For both cat and dog allergens, the evidence for an association between allergen exposure and the development of asthma is insufficient.

An atopic child who has asthma and is sensitized to cat or dog allergen should not live with the respective pet in the home. Pet removal reduces airway responsiveness in those who have pet allergic asthma [64]. Once a pet has been removed, allergen levels in settled dust fall to those seen in homes without cats over 4 to 6 months [65]. Levels fall more rapidly if extensive environmental controls are undertaken, such as removal of carpets, upholstered furniture, and other reservoirs, as well as thorough and repeated cleaning. Cat allergen may persist in mattresses for years after a cat has been removed from a home [66], so the purchase of new bedding or impermeable encasements is recommended also. Because so many sensitized patients are unwilling to remove a pet, many compromise measures have been suggested. The use of high-efficiency particulate air (HEPA) filters and vacuum cleaners results in short-term reductions in airborne cat and dog allergen levels but no change in settled dust allergen concentrations [67–71]. No studies to date show an effect of air filters on disease activity [72], although one study demonstrates a reduction in airway responsiveness without change in any other clinical measure [73].

Rodent (mouse and rat)

Rodent allergens, like cat and dog allergens, are carried on particles that are small and remain airborne [74]. They are primarily excreted in the urine and serve as pheromone-binding proteins [75]. Most studies to date have focused on Mus m 1, the major mouse allergen, which is detectable in settled dust in 82% of homes in the United States and 95% of inner-city homes, with highest levels typically found in the kitchen [76,77]. Mouse allergen levels are higher in homes with reported rodent or cockroach problems [76], but allergen also is found commonly in homes without evidence of mouse infestation [77,78]. One study has measured airborne mouse allergen in inner-city homes, showing that levels in many homes are similar to those found in some occupational settings [74]. Rat n 1, the major rat allergen, is detectable in 33% of inner-city homes [79].

There are data to support a relationship between mouse allergen exposure and skin test sensitization. In inner-city children who have asthma, elevated kitchen mouse allergen levels are associated with a higher rate of mouse sensitization [80]. In suburban asthmatic children, the risk of mouse skin test sensitivity also increases with increasing bedroom exposure to mouse allergen [81]. In contrast, a study of rat allergen has found that sensitization is not more common when allergen is detectable in the home [79].

Although the connection between laboratory rodent exposure and asthma morbidity in sensitized adults has been established, there is, so far, only limited evidence of the impact of mice on childhood asthma. Two studies to date have examined this relationship in the inner-city home environment. One found that exposure to mouse allergen is associated with wheeze in the first year of life [82]. The other showed that, among mouse-sensitized inner-city children, exposure to higher levels of mouse allergen predicts poor asthma control and asthma-related health care use [83]. A study of rat allergen similarly found that rat exposure and sensitization is associated with increased asthma morbidity in inner-city children [79].

Only one clinical trial has assessed the efficacy of rodent allergen reduction methods in the inner-city home setting. A combined 5-month intervention, consisting of filling of holes, vacuuming, cleaning, and use of pesticides and traps, resulted in a significant reduction in mouse allergen levels, but clinical outcomes were not assessed [84].

Conclusions

There is substantial evidence that exposure to various indoor environmental allergens is associated with specific allergic sensitization and increased asthma morbidity. The majority of this research has focused on dust mite, cockroach, and pet allergens, although there is growing evidence that rodent allergens may play an important role in asthma morbidity in inner-city populations. Recommended allergen reduction interventions are summarized in Table 1. Additional studies investigating the efficacy of interventions to reduce indoor allergen exposure and improve asthma outcomes are needed to inform both clinical practice and health policy.

Indoor air pollution and asthma

Exposure to ambient air pollutants has been shown to cause increased airway reactivity, asthma exacerbations, respiratory symptoms and illness,

Table 1
Recommended environmental control practices to reduce indoor allergen exposure

Allergen	Intervention	Strength of recommendation
Dust mite	Install allergen-proof mattress and pillow encasings	+++
	Wash bedding in hot water weekly	+++
	Vacuum carpets frequently	++
	Remove stuffed animals from bed	++
	Remove wall to wall carpeting	++
	Remove draperies and upholstery	++
	Dehumidify	+
	Relocate bedroom from basement	0
	Apply acaracides	0
Cockroach	Exterminate with gel or bait traps (professionally, if possible)	+++
	Appropriately store and discard food	+++
	Clean thoroughly	++
	Repair cracks and holes in structure	+
Cat and dog	Do not bring pet into home or find a new home for existing pet	+++
	Clean home thoroughly after pet removal	+++
	Remove carpets and upholstery after pet removal	++
	Install allergen-proof mattress and pillow encasings	++
	Restrict pet from bedroom	0
	Use HEPA air filter in bedroom	0
Mouse and rat	Exterminate (professionally, if possible)	+++
	Appropriately store and discard food	+++
	Clean thoroughly	++
	Repair cracks and holes in structure	++

decreased lung function, and altered host defense [85–89]. Although Americans spend nearly 90% of their time indoors [90], the focus of scientific investigation for asthma has been on outdoor, rather than indoor, air pollution. Indoor air pollution is a complex mixture of pollutants migrating indoors from ambient air and pollutants generated by unique sources inside the home. Sources of important pollutants relevant to asthma are listed in Table 2. A number of studies have shown that indoor air pollution concentrations can greatly exceed outdoor air concentrations [91]. Although indoor air pollutants and asthma have not been studied thoroughly, research to date suggests that they may play a significant role in asthma morbidity. This article summarizes the findings of the effects of indoor air pollutants (ozone, particulate matter, nitrogen dioxide [NO_2], environmental tobacco smoke, sulfur dioxide [SO_2], and carbon monoxide [CO]) on asthma morbidity.

Table 2
Sources of air pollutants related to asthma incidence and morbidity that are found in indoor air

Pollutant	Source location	Principal sources
Particulate matter	Outdoor and indoor	Numerous sources including combustion (vehicles, power generation, cooking, smoking), resuspended materials (crustal, industrial operations, house dust)
Ozone	Outdoor and indoor	Outdoor: photochemical oxidation, lightning Indoor: photocopiers, ozone generators, welding
Nitrogen dioxide	Outdoor and indoor	Combustion
Sulfur dioxide	Outdoor	Combustion
Environmental tobacco smoke	Indoor	Smoking
Carbon monoxide	Outdoor and indoor	Combustion

Ozone

Ambient ozone is the main contributor to indoor ozone levels; therefore, indoor levels of ozone are related directly to outdoor levels and show significant seasonal variability [91]. Indoor sources of ozone are uncommon but include ionizers or ozone generators, which are sold as air-freshening or air-cleaning devices, and xerographic copy machines found in offices or schools [15]. In addition, among parents working at home, there may be more in-house use of xerographic copy equipment. Epidemiologic studies of ambient ozone and experimental studies show a significant association with asthma-related morbidity, including increases in symptoms, health care use, airway inflammation, and decreases in lung function [89,92–95]. The effect of indoor ozone levels on asthma morbidity has not been well studied. Similarly, the benefits of indoor ozone reduction on asthma morbidity are unknown; however, because ozone is a highly reactive gas, concentrations are generally much lower indoors than outdoors, even in peak ozone season, and evidence suggests that indoor ozone levels may be reduced by keeping windows and doors closed [96]. Furthermore, ozone-generating "air cleaners," "air filters," "air purifiers," and similar equipment should be avoided in the homes of patients who have asthma.

Particulate matter

Particulate matter consists of solid and liquid particles that are suspended in the air. The Environmental Protection Agency regulates two size fractions of airborne particulate matter, $PM_{2.5}$ and PM_{10} (those with aerodynamic diameters <2.5 and <10 μm, respectively). In addition to size, $PM_{2.5}$ and PM_{10} are distinguished by source of generation, with $PM_{2.5}$ produced by agglomeration in combustion processes and PM_{10} produced by comminution (ie, pulverization or fractionization) and resuspension processes. Smoking is a major source of indoor particulate matter; additional sources include cooking and combustion sources such as wood-burning stoves and fireplaces. Larger particles also can be aerosolized by cleaning and other household activities. These larger particles may contain animal allergens and other materials present in reservoir dust inside a home (pesticides, lead, mold spores, and other matter). Studies consistently show an association between elevated outdoor levels of particulate matter and asthma morbidity [97–99]. The few studies that have examined the effects of indoor particulate matter suggest that there is a relationship between indoor levels and asthma outcomes. In particular, indoor particulate matter has been shown to be inversely associated with lung function among children who have asthma [100,101], and $PM_{2.5}$ originating from indoor sources may be more potent per unit mass in decreasing lung function than outdoor-derived particulate matter [101]. Furthermore, a 10-$\mu g/m^3$ increase in indoor $PM_{2.5}$ exposure was associated with a 4.1 ppb increase in exhaled nitric oxide levels, a marker of airway inflammation, in asthmatic children not receiving inhaled corticosteroid medication [101]. Although evidence suggests that particulate matter is related to altered lung function and increased airway inflammation, additional studies are needed to understand the components of indoor particulate matter most associated with asthma as well as the overall impact on asthma exacerbations and asthma-related health care use. Early studies suggest that HEPA filters are effective in lowering concentrations of indoor particulate matter in homes of children who have asthma and may have a modest effect in reducing asthma morbidity [102,103]. Comprehensive strategies of reduction of particulate matter, including source modification, ventilation, and HEPA filter placement, are needed to elucidate better the potential benefit of these strategies on asthma health.

Nitrogen dioxide

NO_2, a common ambient air pollutant, is a product of high-temperature combustion with many potential indoor sources including gas stoves, space heaters, furnaces, and fireplaces. There is limited but suggestive evidence of an association between the use of gas appliances and increased risk of respiratory symptoms in children who have asthma [104,105]. Gas appliances also may confer an additional risk of respiratory symptoms in addition to their effects on measured NO_2 concentrations. For example, gas stoves may increase other indoor air pollutants, such as nitrous acid, which may have adverse effects on respiratory health [104]. Studies specifically investigating the effect of measured indoor NO_2 levels on asthma morbidity have been inconsistent. Some studies have not shown an association between indoor NO_2 levels and asthma morbidity [106]; however, an increasing number of studies have shown a positive association. Increases in indoor NO_2 concentrations increased the likelihood and frequency of asthma symptoms, including wheeze, chest tightness, breathlessness, and daytime and nighttime asthma attacks in two recent studies in asthmatic children [107,108]. NO_2 exposure also has been shown to impair host resistance to respiratory viruses and bacteria through reduction of bacterial clearance and impaired innate immunity [109–111], with higher personal NO_2 exposure increasing the severity of virus-induced asthma exacerbations, measured by symptom severity and peak flow reduction [112]. General control strategies include source modification and ventilation. A randomized, controlled trial studying the effects of reducing NO_2 in schools by replacing unflued gas heaters with flued gas or electric heaters showed a reduction in mean indoor NO_2 concentrations from 47.0 ppb to 15.5 ppb with a concordant decrease in asthma symptoms (difficulty breathing: relative risk [RR], 0.41; 95% confidence interval [CI], 0.07–0.98; chest tightness: RR, 0.45; 95% CI, 0.25–0.81; asthma attacks: RR, 0.39; 95% CI, 0.17–0.93) in schoolchildren [113].

Environmental tobacco smoke

The effect of environmental tobacco smoke or "passive smoking" on asthma has been studied extensively. A significant number of children are exposed to environmental tobacco smoke [114], and there is sufficient evidence to suggest a causal relationship between exposure to environmental tobacco smoke and asthma incidence and morbidity in infants and preschool-aged children. There is, however, limited or insufficient evidence for similar relationships in older, school-aged children [15]. Several studies have linked maternal smoking in utero to decreased lung function, recurrent wheeze in infants, and the incidence of childhood asthma [115–118]. Similarly, postnatal exposure to environmental tobacco smoke has been linked to increased asthma incidence and prevalence [119,120]. A meta-analysis showed the pooled odds ratio for asthma prevalence from 14 case-control studies was 1.37 (95% CI, 1.15–1.64) if either parent smoked [121]. In addition to increased asthma prevalence, exposure to high levels of environmental tobacco smoke has been linked convincingly to increased disease severity among children who have asthma. Specifically, environmental tobacco smoke has been associated with decreased lung function and increased airway inflammation, daytime and nocturnal symptoms, exacerbations, health care use, and intubations [119,122–126]. Smoking is a significant source of indoor particulate matter. In addition, a recent study found that the average concentrations of $PM_{2.5}$ and PM_{10} were 33 to 54 $\mu g/m^3$ greater in households with smokers than in nonsmoking households, with each cigarette smoked adding 1.0 $\mu g/m^3$ to indoor particulate matter concentrations [91]. There is substantial evidence suggesting that avoiding environmental tobacco smoke can result in improved asthma outcomes; however, studies of the effectiveness of interventions attempting to reduce exposure to environmental tobacco smoke show relatively small differences in maternal smoking and in the number of cigarettes smoked in the home [127,128].

To the authors' knowledge, there is no evidence regarding the degree of reduction in exposure to environmental tobacco smoke that can be achieved through ventilation and air cleaning in the homes of smokers who continue to smoke indoors.

Sulfur dioxide

SO_2 is an ambient air pollutant formed mainly when coal or oil containing high levels of sulfur is burned. Indoor sources are not common and include fossil-fuel appliances and furnaces; therefore, personal SO_2 exposure results mainly from ambient air pollution [129]. Because SO_2 is adsorbed rapidly onto household surfaces, the concentration indoors is usually much less than outdoor concentrations. One study indicated that unvented kerosene heaters can produce elevated SO_2 concentrations indoors [130]. Experimental studies suggest that SO_2 can cause decreased lung function in exercising adults who have asthma [131–133]. To the authors' knowledge, no studies have investigated the effects of indoor SO_2 on asthma outcomes. Indirect evidence has been inconclusive also. Using coal for cooking or heating in homes has been found to increase the incidence of asthma in children in a 7-year prospective study [134]; however, a lower prevalence of asthma has been found in other studies [134–136]. The potential role of indoor SO_2 in asthma merits further investigation.

Carbon monoxide

CO is also an ambient air pollutant formed as a product of incomplete combustion. CO concentrations may be elevated in homes with smokers or with gas appliances such as natural gas fireplaces and gas stoves [137]. The most widely recognized adverse effect of CO is the impairment of the oxygen-carrying capacity of hemoglobin. Several studies have shown adverse health effects of ambient CO exposure in children who have asthma [94,138]; however, a significant amount of personal CO exposure may occur in indoor environments [139]. Although elevated CO concentrations in 14 suburban homes with operating kerosene heaters were not associated with altered lung function in healthy residents [130], the effects of elevated indoor CO levels on individuals who have asthma, who may be more susceptible to the effects of CO, are unknown.

Conclusions

There is growing recognition of the importance of the indoor environment in asthma. Specifically, an increasing body of evidence suggests that indoor pollutants contribute to asthma morbidity. The amount of research on indoor air pollution and asthma is small compared with ambient pollutants. Experimental and epidemiologic studies, however, suggest that pollutants, such as NO_2 and ozone, may potentiate the effect of allergen exposure in atopic individuals [140]. More detailed epidemiologic studies comprehensively evaluating the indoor pollutants and allergen exposures are warranted to investigate this interaction further. Although source control seems to be the most reliable method of reducing exposure, additional studies investigating the efficacy of interventions to reduce indoor pollutants and improve asthma outcomes are necessary.

References

[1] Crain EF, Weiss KB, Bijur PE, et al. An estimate of the prevalence of asthma and wheezing among inner-city children. Pediatrics 1994;94:356–62.
[2] Weiss KB, Wagener DK. Changing patterns of asthma mortality: identifying target populations at high risk. J Am Med Assoc 1990;264:1683–7.
[3] Gergen PJ, Weiss KB. Epidemiology of asthma. In: Busse WW, Holgate ST, editors. Asthma and rhinitis. Boston: Blackwell Scientific Publications; 1995. p. 15–31.
[4] Evans R III, Mullaly DI, Wilson RW, et al. National trends in the morbidity and mortality of asthma in the United States. Chest 1987;91:74S–86S.
[5] Peat JK, Britton, Salome CM, et al. Bronchial hyperresponsiveness in two populations of Australian school children: III. Effect of exposure to environmental allergens. Clin Allergy 1987;17:291–300.
[6] Burrows B, Martinez FD, Halonen M, et al. Association of asthma with serum IgE levels and skin-test reactivity to allergens. N Engl J Med 1989;320(5):271–7.
[7] Kang BC, Johnson J, Veres-Torner C. Atopic profile of inner-city asthma with a comparative analysis on the cockroach-sensitive and ragweed-sensitive subgroups. J Allergy Clin Immunol 1993;92:802–11.
[8] Unger L. The house-dust mite. Ann Allergy 1967;25(10):598–9.
[9] Tovey ER, Chapman MD, Wells CW, et al. The distribution of dust mite allergen in the houses of patients with asthma. Am Rev Respir Dis 1981;124(5):630–5.
[10] Tovey E, Marks G. Methods and effectiveness of environmental control. J Allergy Clin Immunol 1999;103:179–91.
[11] Wickman M, Nordvall SL, Pershagen G, et al. Sensitization to domestic mites in a cold temperate region. Am Rev Respir Dis 1993;148:58–62.
[12] Platts-Mills TAE, Hayden ML, Chapman MD, et al. Seasonal variation in dust mite and grass pollen allergens in dust from the houses of patients with asthma. J Allergy Clin Immunol 1987;79:781–91.
[13] Kuehr J, Frischer T, Meinert R, et al. Mite allergen exposure is a risk for the incidence of specific sensitization. J Allergy Clin Immunol 1994;94:44–52.
[14] Huss K, Adkinson NF Jr, Eggleston PA, et al. House dust mite and cockroach exposure are strong risk factors for positive allergy skin test responses in the Childhood Asthma Management Program. J Allergy Clin Immunol 2001;107(1):48–54.
[15] Institute of Medicine Committee on the Assessment of Asthma and Indoor Air. Clearing the air: asthma and indoor air exposures. Washington, DC: National academy press; 2000.
[16] Sporik R, Holgate ST, Platts-Mills TA, et al. Exposure to house-dust mite allergen (Der p I) and the development of asthma in childhood. A prospective study. N Engl J Med 1990; 323(8):502–7.
[17] Shaver JR, Zangrilli JG, Cho SK, et al. Kinetics of the development and recovery of the lung from IgE-mediated inflammation: dissociation of pulmonary eosinophilia, lung injury, and eosinophil-active cytokines. Am J Respir Crit Care Med 1997;155(2):442–8.
[18] Eggleston PA, Bush RK. Environmental allergen avoidance: an overview. J Allergy Clin Immunol 2001;107(3 suppl):S403–5.

[19] Ehnert B, Lau-Schadendorf S, Weber A, et al. Reducing domestic exposure to dust mite allergen reduces bronchial hyperreactivity in sensitive children with asthma. J Allergy Clin Immunol 1992;90:135–8.

[20] Walshaw MJ, Evans CC. Allergen avoidance in house dust mite sensitive adult asthma. Q J Med 1986;226:199–215.

[21] Carswell F, Birmingham K, Oliver J, et al. The respiratory effects of reduction of mite allergen in the bedrooms of asthmatic children-a double-blind controlled trial. Clin Exp Allergy 1996;26:386–96.

[22] van der Heide S, Kauffman HF, Dubois AEJ, et al. Allergen-avoidance measures in homes of house-dust-mite-allergic asthmatic patients: effects of acaracides and mattress encasing. Allergy 1997;52:921–7.

[23] Shapiro GG, Wighton TG, Chin T, et al. House dust mite avoidance for children with asthma in homes of low-income families. J Allergy Clin Immunol 1999;103:1069–74.

[24] Htut T, Higenbottam TW, Gill GW, et al. Eradication of house dust mite from homes of atopic asthmatic subjects: a double-blind trial. J Allergy Clin Immunol 2001;107:55–60.

[25] Frederick JM, Warner JO, Jessop WJ, et al. Effect of a bed covering system in children with asthma and house dust mite hypersensitivity. Eur Respir J 1997;10:361–6.

[26] Vaughan JW, McLaughlin TE, Perzanowski MS, et al. Evaluation of materials used for bedding encasement: effect of pore size in blocking cat and dust mite allergen. J Allergy Clin Immunol 1999;103:227–31.

[27] Woodcock A, Forster L, Matthews E, et al. Control of exposure to mite allergen and allergen-impermeable bed covers for adults with asthma. N Engl J Med 2003;349(3):225–36.

[28] McDonald LG, Tovey E. The role of water temperature and laundry procedures in reducing house dust mite populations and allergen content of bedding. J Allergy Clin Immunol 1992;90:599–608.

[29] Vandehove T, Soler M, Birnbaum J, et al. Effect of dry cleaning on the mite allergen levels in blankets. Allergy 1993;48:264–6.

[30] Mason K, Riley G, Siebers R, et al. Hot tumble drying and mite survival in duvets. J Allergy Clin Immunol 1999;104:499–500.

[31] Munir AK, Einarsson R, Dreborg SK. Vacuum cleaning decreases the levels of mite allergens in house dust. Pediatr Allergy Immunol 1993;4:136–43.

[32] Sporik R, Hill DJ, Thompson PJ, et al. The Melbourne house dust mite study: long-term efficacy of house dust mite reduction strategies. J Allergy Clin Immunol 1998;101:451–6.

[33] Woodfolk JA, Hayden M, Miller J, et al. Chemical treatment of carpets to reduce allergen: a detailed study of the effects of tannic acid on indoor allergens. J Allergy Clin Immunol 1994;94:19–26.

[34] Hayden ML, Rose G, Diduch KB, et al. Benzylbenzoate moist powder: investigation of acaricidal activity in cultures and reduction of dust mite allergens in carpets. J Allergy Clin Immunol 1992;89:536–45.

[35] Arlian LG, Neal JS, Morgan MS, et al. Reducing relative humidity in homes is a practical way to control house dust mites and their allergens in homes in temperate climates. J Allergy Clin Immunol 2001;107:99–104.

[36] Custovic A, Taggart SCO, Kennaugh JH, et al. Portable dehumidifiers in the control of house dust mites and mite allergens. Clin Exp Allergy 1994;25:312–6.

[37] Eggleston PA, Arruda LK. Ecology and elimination of cockroaches and allergens in the home. J Allergy Clin Immunol 2001;107:S422–9.

[38] Kattan M, Mitchell H, Eggleston P, et al. Characteristics of inner-city children with asthma: the National Cooperative Inner-City Asthma Study. Pediatr Pulmonol 1997;24:253–62.

[39] Eggleston PA, Rosenstreich D, Lynn H, et al. Relationship of indoor allergen exposure to skin test sensitivity in inner-city children with asthma. J Allergy Clin Immunol 1998;102(4 Pt 1):563–70.

[40] Matsui EC, Wood RA, Rand C, et al. Cockroach allergen exposure and sensitization in suburban middle-class children with asthma. J Allergy Clin Immunol 2003;112(1):87–92.

[41] Sarpong SB, Hamilton RG, Eggleston PA, et al. Socioeconomic status and race as risk factors for cockroach allergen exposure and sensitization in children with asthma. J Allergy Clin Immunol 1996;97(6):1393–401.
[42] Rosenstreich DL, Eggleston PA, Kattan M, et al, for the National Cooperative Inner City Asthma Study. The role of cockroach allergy and exposure to cockroach allergen in causing morbidity among inner-city children with asthma. N Engl J Med 1997;336:1356–63.
[43] Gold DR, Burge HA, Carey V, et al. Predictors of repeated wheeze in the first year of life: the relative roles of cockroach, birth weight, acute lower respiratory illness, and maternal smoking. Am J Respir Crit Care Med 1999;160(1):227–36.
[44] Eggleston PA, Wood RA, Rand C, et al. Removal of cockroach allergen from inner city homes. J Allergy Clin Immunol 1999;104:842–6.
[45] Reid BL, Bennett GW. Apartments: field trials of abamectin bait formulations. Insecticide Acaracide Tests 1989;17:4.
[46] Wright CG, Dupree NE. Single family dwellings: evaluation of insecticides for controlling German cockroaches. Insecticide Acaracide Tests 1988;15:355.
[47] Bennett GW, Owens JM, Corrigan RM. Trumans scientific guide to pest control operations. 4th edition. Duluth (MN): Edgell Communications; 1988.
[48] Arbes SJ Jr, Sever M, Mehta J, et al. Abatement of cockroach allergens (Bla g 1 and Bla g 2) in low-income urban housing: month 12 results. J Allergy Clin Immunol 2004;113:109–14.
[49] Gergen PJ, Mortimer KM, Eggleston PA, et al. Results of the National Cooperative Inner City Asthma Study (NCICAS) environmental intervention to reduce cockroach allergen exposure in inner-city homes. J Allergy Clin Immunol 1999;103(3 Pt 1):501–6.
[50] Morgan WJ, Crain EF, Gruchalla RS, et al. Results of a home-based environmental intervention among urban children with asthma. N Engl J Med 2004;351:1068–80.
[51] Evans R, Gergen PJ, Mitchell H, et al. A randomized clinical trial to reduce asthma morbidity among inner-city children: results of the National Cooperative Inner-City Asthma Study. J Pediatr 1999;135(3):332–8.
[52] Custovic A, Green R, Fletcher A, et al. Aerodynamic properties of the major dog allergen, Can f 1: distribution in homes, concentration, and particle size of allergen in air. Am J Respir Crit Care Med 1997;155:94–8.
[53] Almqvist C, Larrson PH, Egmar A-C, et al. School as a risk environment for children allergic to cats and a site for transfer of cat allergen to homes. J Allergy Clin Immunol 1999;103:1012–7.
[54] Custovic A, Fletcher A, Pickering CAC, et al. Domestic allergens in public places III: house dust mite, cat, dog and cockroach allergens in British hospitals. Clin Exp Allergy 1998;28:53–9.
[55] Bollinger ME, Eggleston PA, Flanagan E, et al. Cat antigen in homes with and without cats may induce allergic symptoms. J Allergy Clin Immunol 1996;97(4):907–14.
[56] Wood RA, Eggleston PA, Ingemann L, et al. Antigenic analysis of household dust samples. Am Rev Respir Dis 1998;137:358–63.
[57] Simpson A, Custovic A. Pets and the development of allergic sensitization. Curr Allergy Asthma Rep 2005;5(3):212–20.
[58] Almqvist C, Egmar AC, Hedlin G, et al. Direct and indirect exposure to pets—risk of sensitization and asthma at 4 years in a birth cohort. Clin Exp Allergy 2003;33(9):1190–7.
[59] Henriksen AH, Holmen TL, Bjermer L. Sensitization and exposure to pet allergens in asthmatics versus non-asthmatics with allergic rhinitis. Respir Med 2001;95(2):122–9.
[60] Norman PS, Ohman JL, Long AA, et al. Treatment of cat allergy with T-cell reactive peptides. Am J Respir Crit Care Med 1996;154(6 Pt 1):1623–8.
[61] Sicherer SH, Wood RA, Eggleston PA. Determinants of airway responses to cat allergen: comparison of environmental challenge to quantitative nasal and bronchial allergen challenge. J Allergy Clin Immunol 1997;99(6 Pt 1):798–805.
[62] Hedlin G, Heilborn H, Lilja G, et al. Long-term follow-up of patients treated with a three-year course of cat or dog immunotherapy. J Allergy Clin Immunol 1995;96(6 Pt 1):879–85.

[63] Valovirta E, Koivikko A, Vanto T, et al. Immunotherapy in allergy to dog: a double-blind clinical study. Ann Allergy 1984;53(1):85–8.

[64] Shirai T, Matsui T, Suzuki K, et al. Effect of pet removal on pet allergic asthma. Chest 2005; 127(5):1565–71.

[65] Wood RA, Chapman MD, Adkinson NF Jr, et al. The effect of cat removal on Fel D 1 content in household dust samples. J Allergy Clin Immunol 1989;83:730–4.

[66] Van der Brempt X, Charpin D, Haddi E, et al. Cat removal and Fel d 1 levels in mattresses. J Allergy Clin Immunol 1991;87:595–6.

[67] De Blay F, Chapman MD, Platts-Mills TAE. Airborne cat allergen (Fel d 1): environmental control with the cat in situ. Am Rev Respir Dis 1991;143:1334–9.

[68] Avner DB, Perzanowski MS, Platts-Mills TAE, et al. Evaluation of different techniques for washing cats: quantitation of allergen removed from the cat and effect on airborne Fel d 1. J Allergy Clin Immunol 1997;100:307–12.

[69] Green R, Simpson A, Custovic A, et al. The effect of air filtration on airborne dog allergen. Allergy 1999;54:484–8.

[70] Gore RB, Bishop S, Durrell L, et al. Air filtration units in homes with cats: can they reduce personal exposure to cat allergen? Clin Exp Allergy 2003;33:765–9.

[71] Francis H, Fletcher G, Anthony C, et al. Effects of air filters in homes of asthmatic adults sensitized and exposed to pet allergens. Clin Exp Allergy 2003;33:101–5.

[72] Wood RA, Flanagan E, Van Natta M, et al. A placebo-controlled trial of a HEPA air cleaner in the treatment of cat allergy. Am J Respir Crit Care Med 1998;158:115–20.

[73] Van der Heide S, van Aalderen WMC, Kauffman HF, et al. Clinical effects of air cleaners in homes of children sensitized to pet allergens. J Allergy Clin Immunol 1999;104: 447–51.

[74] Matsui EC, Simons E, Rand C, et al. Airborne mouse allergen in the homes of inner city children with asthma. J Allergy Clin Immunol 2005;115:358–63.

[75] Schumacher MJ. Clinically relevant allergens from laboratory and domestic small animals. N Engl Reg Allergy Proc 1987;8(4):225–31.

[76] Cohn RD, Arbes ST Jr, Yin M, et al. National prevalence and exposure risk for mouse allergen in US households. J Allergy Clin Immunol 2004;113:1167–71.

[77] Phipatanakul W, Eggleston PA, Wright EC, et al. Mouse allergen I. The prevalence of mouse allergen in inner-city homes. The National Cooperative Inner-City Asthma Study. J Allergy Clin Immunol 2000;106(6):1070–4.

[78] Chew GL, Perzanowski MS, Miller RL, et al. Distribution and determinants of mouse allergen exposure in low-income New York City apartments. Environ Health Perspect 2003; 111(10):1348–51.

[79] Perry T, Matsui E, Merriman B, et al. The prevalence of rat allergen in inner-city homes and its relationship to sensitization and asthma morbidity. J Allergy Clin Immunol 2003;112(2): 346–52.

[80] Phipatanakul W, Eggleston PA, Wright EC, et al. Mouse allergen II. The relationship of mouse allergen exposure to mouse sensitization and asthma morbidity in inner-city children with asthma. J Allergy Clin Immunol 2000;106(6):1075–80.

[81] Matsui EC, Wood RA, Rand C, et al. Mouse allergen exposure and mouse skin test sensitivity in suburban, middle-class children with asthma. J Allergy Clin Immunol 2004;113(5): 910–5.

[82] Phipatanakul W, Celedon JC, Sredl DL, et al. Mouse exposure and wheeze in the first year of life. Ann Allergy Asthma Immunol 2005;94(5):593–9.

[83] Matsui EC, Eggleston PA, Buckley TJ, et al. Household mouse allergen exposure and asthma morbidity in inner-city preschool children. Ann Allergy Asthma Immunol 2006; 97(4):514–20.

[84] Phipatanakul W, Cronin B, Wood RA, et al. Effect of environmental intervention on mouse allergen levels in homes of inner-city Boston children with asthma. Ann Allergy Asthma Immunol 2004;92(4):420–5.

[85] Bates DV, Sizto R. Air pollution and hospital admissions in Southern Ontario: the acid summer haze effect. Environ Res 1987;43(2):317–31.

[86] Lioy PJ, Vollmuth TA, Lippmann M. Persistence of peak flow decrement in children following ozone exposures exceeding the National Ambient Air Quality Standard. J Air Pollut Control Assoc 1985;35(10):1069–71.

[87] Schwartz J, Slater D, Larson TV, et al. Particulate air pollution and hospital emergency room visits for asthma in Seattle. Am Rev Respir Dis 1993;147(4):826–31.

[88] Peters A, Dockery DW, Heinrich J, et al. Short-term effects of particulate air pollution on respiratory morbidity in asthmatic children. Eur Respir J 1997;10(4):872–9.

[89] Kim JJ. American Academy of Pediatrics Committee on Environmental Health. Ambient air pollution: health hazards to children. Pediatrics 2004;114(6):1699–707.

[90] Klepeis NE, Nelson WC, Ott WR, et al. The National Human Activity Pattern Survey (NHAPS): a resource for assessing exposure to environmental pollutants. J Expo Anal Environ Epidemiol 2001;11(3):231–52.

[91] Breysse PN, Buckley TJ, Williams D, et al. Indoor exposures to air pollutants and allergens in the homes of asthmatic children in inner-city Baltimore. Environ Res 2005;98(2):167–76.

[92] Mortimer KM, Neas LM, Dockery DW, et al. The effect of air pollution on inner-city children with asthma. Eur Respir J 2002;19(4):699–705.

[93] Graham DE, Koren HS. Biomarkers of inflammation in ozone-exposed humans. Comparison of the nasal and bronchoalveolar lavage. Am Rev Respir Dis 1990;142(1):152–6.

[94] Lin M, Chen Y, Burnett RT, et al. Effect of short-term exposure to gaseous pollution on asthma hospitalisation in children: a bi-directional case-crossover analysis. J Epidemiol Community Health 2003;57(1):50–5.

[95] Ross MA, Persky VW, Scheff PA, et al. Effect of ozone and aeroallergens on the respiratory health of asthmatics. Arch Environ Health 2002;57(6):568–78.

[96] Gold DR, Allen G, Damokosh A, et al. Comparison of outdoor and classroom ozone exposures for school children in Mexico City. J Air Waste Manage Assoc 1996;46(4): 335–42.

[97] Koren HS. Associations between criteria air pollutants and asthma. Environ Health Perspect 1995;103(Suppl 6):235–42.

[98] Delfino RJ, Zeiger RS, Seltzer JM, et al. Association of asthma symptoms with peak particulate air pollution and effect modification by anti-inflammatory medication use. Environ Health Perspect 2002;110(10):A607–17.

[99] Koenig JQ, Larson TV, Hanley QS, et al. Pulmonary function changes in children associated with fine particulate matter. Environ Res 1993;63(1):26–38.

[100] Delfino RJ, Quintana PJ, Floro J, et al. Association of FEV1 in asthmatic children with personal and microenvironmental exposure to airborne particulate matter. Environ Health Perspect 2004;112(8):932–41.

[101] Koenig JQ, Mar TF, Allen RW, et al. Pulmonary effects of indoor- and outdoor-generated particles in children with asthma. Environ Health Perspect 2005;113(4):499–503.

[102] Eggleston PA, Butz A, Rand C, et al. Home environmental intervention in inner-city asthma: a randomized controlled clinical trial. Ann Allergy Asthma Immunol 2005;95(6): 518–24.

[103] Reisman RE, Mauriello PM, Davis GB, et al. A double-blind study of the effectiveness of a high-efficiency particulate air (HEPA) filter in the treatment of patients with perennial allergic rhinitis and asthma. J Allergy Clin Immunol 1990;85(6):1050–7.

[104] Garrett MH, Hooper MA, Hooper BM, et al. Respiratory symptoms in children and indoor exposure to nitrogen dioxide and gas stoves. Am J Respir Crit Care Med 1998;158(3): 891–5.

[105] Ostro BD, Lipsett MJ, Mann JK, et al. Indoor air pollution and asthma. Results from a panel study. Am J Respir Crit Care Med 1994;149(6):1400–6.

[106] Hoek G, Brunekreef B, Meijer R, et al. Indoor nitrogen dioxide pollution and respiratory symptoms of schoolchildren. Int Arch Occup Environ Health 1984;55(1):79–86.

[107] Belanger K, Gent JF, Triche EW, et al. Association of indoor nitrogen dioxide exposure with respiratory symptoms in children with asthma. Am J Respir Crit Care Med 2006; 173(3):297–303.

[108] Smith BJ, Nitschke M, Pilotto LS, et al. Health effects of daily indoor nitrogen dioxide exposure in people with asthma. Eur Respir J 2000;16(5):879–85.

[109] Jakab GJ. Modulation of pulmonary defense mechanisms by acute exposures to nitrogen dioxide. Environ Res 1987;42(1):215–28.

[110] Ehrlich R. Effect of nitrogen dioxide on resistance to respiratory infection. Bacteriol Rev 1966;30(3):604–14.

[111] Frampton MW, Smeglin AM, Roberts NJ Jr, et al. Nitrogen dioxide exposure in vivo and human alveolar macrophage inactivation of influenza virus in vitro. Environ Res 1989; 48(2):179–92.

[112] Chauhan AJ, Inskip HM, Linaker CH, et al. Personal exposure to nitrogen dioxide (NO2) and the severity of virus-induced asthma in children. Lancet 2003;361(9373): 1939–44.

[113] Pilotto LS, Nitschke M, Smith BJ, et al. Randomized controlled trial of unflued gas heater replacement on respiratory health of asthmatic schoolchildren. Int J Epidemiol 2004;33(1): 208–14.

[114] Gergen PJ, Fowler JA, Maurer KR, et al. The burden of environmental tobacco smoke exposure on the respiratory health of children 2 months through 5 years of age in the United States: Third National Health and Nutrition Examination Survey, 1988 to 1994. Pediatrics 1998;101(2):E8.

[115] Infante-Rivard C, Gautrin D, Malo JL, et al. Maternal smoking and childhood asthma. Am J Epidemiol 1999;150(5):528–31.

[116] DiFranza JR, Aligne CA, Weitzman M. Prenatal and postnatal environmental tobacco smoke exposure and children's health. Pediatrics 2004;113(4 Suppl):1007–15.

[117] Lannero E, Wickman M, Pershagen G, et al. Maternal smoking during pregnancy increases the risk of recurrent wheezing during the first years of life (BAMSE). Respir Res 2006;7:3.

[118] Zlotkowska R, Zejda JE. Fetal and postnatal exposure to tobacco smoke and respiratory health in children. Eur J Epidemiol 2005;20(8):719–27.

[119] Martinez FD, Cline M, Burrows B. Increased incidence of asthma in children of smoking mothers. Pediatrics 1992;89(1):21–6.

[120] Sturm JJ, Yeatts K, Loomis D. Effects of tobacco smoke exposure on asthma prevalence and medical care use in North Carolina middle school children. Am J Public Health 2004;94(2):308–13.

[121] Strachan DP, Cook DG. Health effects of passive smoking. 6. Parental smoking and childhood asthma: longitudinal and case-control studies. Thorax 1998;53(3):204–12.

[122] Evans D, Levison MJ, Feldman CH, et al. The impact of passive smoking on emergency room visits of urban children with asthma. Am Rev Respir Dis 1987;135(3):567–72.

[123] LeSon S, Gershwin ME. Risk factors for asthmatic patients requiring intubation. I. Observations in children. J Asthma 1995;32(4):285–94.

[124] Cook DG, Strachan DP. Health effects of passive smoking. 3. Parental smoking and prevalence of respiratory symptoms and asthma in school age children. Thorax 1997;52(12): 1081–94.

[125] Morkjaroenpong V, Rand CS, Butz AM, et al. Environmental tobacco smoke exposure and nocturnal symptoms among inner-city children with asthma. J Allergy Clin Immunol 2002; 110(1):147–53.

[126] Feleszko W, Zawadzka-Krajewska A, Matysiak K, et al. Parental tobacco smoking is associated with augmented IL-13 secretion in children with allergic asthma. J Allergy Clin Immunol 2006;117(1):97–102.

[127] Wilson SR, Yamada EG, Sudhakar R, et al. A controlled trial of an environmental tobacco smoke reduction intervention in low-income children with asthma. Chest 2001;120(5): 1709–22.

[128] Klerman L. Protecting children: reducing their environmental tobacco smoke exposure. Nicotine Tob Res 2004;6(Suppl 2):S239–53.

[129] Lee K, Bartell SM, Paek D. Interpersonal and daily variability of personal exposures to nitrogen dioxide and sulfur dioxide. J Expo Anal Environ Epidemiol 2004;14(2):137–43.

[130] Cooper KR, Alberti RR. Effect of kerosene heater emissions on indoor air quality and pulmonary function. Am Rev Respir Dis 1984;129(4):629–31.

[131] Linn WS, Venet TG, Shamoo DA, et al. Respiratory effects of sulfur dioxide in heavily exercising asthmatics. A dose-response study. Am Rev Respir Dis 1983;127(3):278–83.

[132] Roger LJ, Kehrl HR, Hazucha M, et al. Bronchoconstriction in asthmatics exposed to sulfur dioxide during repeated exercise. J Appl Physiol 1985;59(3):784–91.

[133] Schachter EN, Witek TJ Jr, Beck GJ, et al. Airway effects of low concentrations of sulfur dioxide: dose-response characteristics. Arch Environ Health 1984;39(1):34–42.

[134] Zejda JE, Kowalska M. Risk factors for asthma in school children–results of a seven-year follow-up. Cent Eur J Public Health 2003;11(3):149–54.

[135] Volkmer RE, Ruffin RE, Wigg NR, et al. The prevalence of respiratory symptoms in South Australian preschool children. II. Factors associated with indoor air quality. J Paediatr Child Health 1995;31(2):116–20.

[136] von Mutius E, Illi S, Nicolai T, et al. Relation of indoor heating with asthma, allergic sensitisation, and bronchial responsiveness: survey of children in south Bavaria. BMJ 1996; 312(7044):1448–50.

[137] Dutton SJ, Hannigan MP, Miller SL. Indoor pollutant levels from the use of unvented natural gas fireplaces in Boulder, Colorado. J Air Waste Manage Assoc 2001;51(12):1654–61.

[138] Yu O, Sheppard L, Lumley T, et al. Effects of ambient air pollution on symptoms of asthma in Seattle-area children enrolled in the CAMP study. Environ Health Perspect 2000; 108(12):1209–14.

[139] De Bruin YB, Carrer P, Jantunen M, et al. Personal carbon monoxide exposure levels: contribution of local sources to exposures and microenvironment concentrations in Milan. J Expo Anal Environ Epidemiol 2004;14(4):312–22.

[140] Tunnicliffe WS, Burge PS, Ayres JG. Effect of domestic concentrations of nitrogen dioxide on airway responses to inhaled allergen in asthmatic patients. Lancet 1994;344(8939–8940): 1733–6.

ELSEVIER
SAUNDERS

Pediatr Clin N Am
54 (2007) 121–133

PEDIATRIC CLINICS
OF NORTH AMERICA

Children's Health in the Rural Environment

Debra C. Cherry, MD, MS[a,b,*],
Barbara Huggins, MD[b,c], Karen Gilmore, MPH[a,d]

[a]*Occupational Health Sciences, University of Texas Health Center at Tyler,
11937 US Highway 271, Tyler, TX 75708, USA*
[b]*Southwest Center for Pediatric Environmental Health, 11937 US Highway 271,
Tyler, TX 75708, USA*
[c]*Department of Pediatrics, University of Texas Health Center at Tyler,
11937 US Highway 271, Tyler, TX 75708, USA*
[d]*Southwest Center for Agricultural Health, Injury Prevention, and Education,
University of Texas Health Center at Tyler, 11937 US Highway 271,
Tyler, TX 75708, USA*

Rural children are a diverse group. The definition of "rural" varies widely, with contradictions in classification between government agencies [1,2]. In this article, "rural" has a broad definition, including nonmetropolitan and nonurban residents regardless of involvement with agriculture. Rural residents may be farmers, factory workers, migrant farm workers, retired grandparents, or wealthy professionals. Health risks such as drug abuse, traumatic injuries, chemical and pollutant exposure, excessive television viewing, and poor diet resulting in obesity impact both urban and rural children [3] but actually are exaggerated in the rural population. This article explores differences in the health profiles of rural and urban children and describes facets of the rural environment that especially impact the health of children.

This article was supported in part by the Southwest Center for Pediatric Environmental Health, a component of the Pediatric Environmental Health Specialty Units funded by the Association of Occupational and Environmental Clinics (AOEC) through a cooperative agreement with the Agency for Toxic Substances and Disease Registry (ATSDR) and the Environmental Protection Agency (EPA).

* Corresponding author. Occupational Health Sciences, University of Texas Health Center at Tyler, 11937 US HWY 271, Tyler, TX 75708.

E-mail address: debra.cherry@uthct.edu (D.C. Cherry).

Rural demographics

Although rural children are extremely diverse, some trends emerge from population-based data. Compared with urban children, a larger portion of rural children in the United States are poor and white and have less-educated parents (Table 1) [4]. Rural children engage in a bit more smoking, drinking, and drug use [5,6] than their urban counterparts, but less teen sex (see Table 1) [7,8]. Smokeless tobacco also is popular among rural teens, especially males [2,9]. Methamphetamine abuse is a rampant epidemic in the rural Midwest that impacts children both directly and indirectly [10]. Rural children also have a higher mortality rate than urban children in every age group [6] for a variety of reasons (see Table 1). Special rural populations include migrant farm workers [11] and extremely poor families in South Texas, Appalachia, and parts of the Southwest [4].

Facets of the rural environment that impact children's health

Rural air quality

Although they lack the smog associated with heavy traffic, rural areas sometimes have worse air quality problems. Individuals living in the rural setting may encounter a variety of inhaled organic dusts, including molds and pollens in the air, dusts generated in silos and barns, animal dander, and grain dust [12]. Particulate matter in dry, dusty areas may aggravate asthma or cause pulmonary fibrosis after a period of years, especially if silica is a component [13]. Rural children may encounter toxic gas. For instance, silo filler's disease, characterized by delayed pulmonary edema and

Table 1
Demographics, behavior, and mortality: rural versus urban children

	Rural (%)	Urban (%)
Children living in poverty [4]	21	18
White race[a] [4]	80–89[a]	44–71[a]
Parents with 1+ years college [4]	47	57
Teens reporting daily smoking [5]	19	11
Binge drinking, 10th graders [6]	26	21
Illicit drug use, 10th graders [6]	22	19
High school teens (grades 9–12) who report ever having sexual intercourse [7,8]	Rural Illinois: 33 Median, 29 states: 43.6	Chicago: 58 Median, 17 urban areas: 48.1
Mortality per 100,000 teens [6]	87	62

[a] *Additional data from* US Census Bureau, American fact finder data query, census 2000 summary file 2 (sf-2), pct-2 urban and rural (universe: total population), race = white alone and the Brookings Institution Center on Urban and Metropolitan Policy. Racial changes in the nation's largest cities: evidence from the 2000 census; April 1, 2001. Available at: http://www.brook.edu/es/urban/census/citygrowth.htm; accessed June 27, 2006.

pneumonitis, may result from unintentional exposure to nitrogen dioxide accumulating in the silo [14]. Concentrated animal feedlot operations (CAFOs) release emissions such as hydrogen sulfide, ammonia, particulates, and bioaerosols and lead to increased complaints of respiratory illness, diarrhea, headache, and burning eyes in those who live nearby [5]. The most prevalent air pollution risk for rural children is exposure to environmental tobacco smoke indoors, because the rate of cigarette smoking is higher in rural areas (33% prevalence of smokers, versus 27% in large metropolitan areas) [15].

The impact of rural living on the respiratory health of children is complex. Despite some unique exposure risks, rural residence has been associated with less cough, less asthma, and better tolerance of chronic obstructive pulmonary disease than urban residence [16]. Life on the farm in early childhood seems to prevent the development of asthma later in life [17–19], particularly when combined with maternal exposure to farm animals during pregnancy and lactation [20]. Rural residence alone is not a risk factor for respiratory disease but rather is an indication for considering special environmental exposures when respiratory disease is present.

Water quality in rural areas

The United States has one of the safest drinking water supplies in the world [21]. In rural areas, however, municipal water may be unavailable. More rural families get their water from wells, and the well owner alone is responsible for ensuring the quality of the well water. Occasionally, well water is contaminated by leaking underground storage tanks, microbes, pesticides, or other chemicals [22]. Just as they lack municipal water, many families lack municipal sewage and use a septic system instead. If not properly maintained, septic tanks are susceptible to overflowing and contaminating surface water or well water. The density of septic tanks in an area has been correlated with the incidence of diarrhea in children [23].

Agriculture is a source of pollution for 48% of river miles classified as impaired by the Environmental Protection Agency [24]. CAFOs are a particular threat to rivers and lakes in rural areas, releasing pollutants such as nitrogen and phosphorus, organic matter, sediments, pathogens, heavy metals, hormones, antibiotics, and ammonia to the waterways. These pollutants may cause toxic algal blooms, fish kills, and outbreaks of pathogens such as cryptosporidium [25]. Children living near CAFOs should take special precautions not to drink or swim in contaminated water.

Well water is not supplemented with fluoride, nor are many rural municipal water systems [2]. Rural children tend to have more sugar in their diets [26], less access to dentists [2], and more dental caries [27] than their urban counterparts. Therefore, rural children may have a particular need for fluoride supplementation to prevent tooth decay.

Animal safety and firearms

Injury from encountering large animals represents a significant health risk for rural children, especially those who live on or visit farms. Horses, bulls, and cows are the animals most often associated with children's injuries [28,29]. Chores such as feeding animals or cleaning out livestock pens may lead to injury. Farm animals may knock down, step on, kick, or trample children without provocation [30], causing injuries to the torso, long bones, or craniofacial structures. In addition, zoonotic disease such as bird flu may spread from livestock to children [31]. Approaching animals safely and washing hands thoroughly after touching animals are keys to prevention of injury and transmission of diseases. Another prevention alternative is to eliminate contact with animals by prohibiting access to the farm worksite, installing passive safety barriers, and designating safe play areas on farms away from animals [32].

Target shooting and hunting are common avocations in rural areas. Firearm injuries that occur while hunting, sport shooting, or target shooting account for a substantial portion of all fatal and nonfatal unintentional injuries in children [33,34]. The typical victim of an unintentional firearm injury is a young male with a self-inflicted wound to a limb [35]. In a random telephone survey in northeast Ohio, only 12% (15/122) of gun owners with children between the ages of 5 and 15 years stored their guns locked and unloaded, a habit correlated with higher education and income but not with urban or rural residence [36]. Most firearm accidents are completely preventable with better gun safety habits.

Rural traffic and motor vehicle–related injuries

Motor vehicle crashes are the leading cause of unintentional death in the rural population in some states [34,37]. Using data from the Federal Highway Administration from 1998 to 2000, Clark and Cushing [38] reported that population density was a moderately strong predictor of rural traffic mortality rates; the rate of deaths per 100 million vehicle miles traveled was inversely proportional to population density. In addition, Zwerling and colleagues [39], using national databases, found that the incidence of fatal crashes was more than two times higher in rural than in urban areas. Explanations for this troubling and persistent statistic include lack of seat belt use [40,41], poor road conditions, and delayed access to pediatric trauma care [42].

Another motor vehicle risk unique to rural areas is the recreational use of all terrain vehicles (ATVs). The American Academy of Pediatrics policy statement discourages ATV use for children younger than 16 years of age [43], but ATV injuries and deaths in young children are on the rise [44]. Of the 6313 deaths caused by ATVs between 1982 and 2003, one third of the riders who were killed or injured were younger than 16 years. Head injuries, clothesline injuries to the neck and face, and spinal cord transections are common causes of death, permanent disability, and serious injuries for children involved in ATV mishaps [45].

Rural bodies of water and drowning

Drowning deaths in youth living in rural areas are as common as motor vehicle–related deaths and are second only to occupational fatalities on the farm [46]. An average of thirty-two farm drowning deaths occur in youth every year [47], accounting for one third of all farm deaths in this population. Although the bodies of water in rural areas in which drowning occurs may differ from those in more urban areas (lakes and ponds versus swimming pools), the reasons for drowning are consistent with the causes of unintentional drowning in more urban populations. These include absence of adult supervision, lack of effective barriers between the body of water and the child, and the stage of the child's development [48]. Unfortunately, as with many cases of injury occurring in rural areas, the drowning injuries of rural children are more likely to be fatal. In fact, Nixon and colleagues [49] found that the survival rates for unsupervised children who lose consciousness in fresh water are site dependent. Only 21% of such potential victims survived after losing consciousness in rivers and creeks, compared with 65% of those involved in potential drowning incidents in their own backyard. Because of the prevalence of drowning in rural areas, emphasis on education for parents and children regarding prevention, provision of resources for available safety devices, and potential regulations to provide safe play areas for children should be developed [50].

Rural lifestyle and obesity

Although it would be tempting to assume that children living in rural areas would have many opportunities for getting plenty of activity and for eating healthy foods, this is not the case. Investigators from several areas of the United States have found a higher prevalence of obesity in adults and children living in rural areas [51–55]. The reasons are not complicated. As in most cases, diet and activity are the key determinants. Surprisingly, the dietary habits of rural children often mirror those of their urban counterparts. Evidence of health disparities of children living in rural areas was discovered by Davy and colleagues [52] when they examined the nutritional intake of middle school–aged children in rural Mississippi. They determined that the knowledge of these children regarding the importance of diet and exercise in preventing cardiovascular disease was poor. These children also were noted to have saturated fat and sodium intake that exceeded recommended levels. In addition, their intake of calcium, fruits, and vegetables was inadequate. More than one third reported drinking 12 oz of soda daily.

The Behavioral Risk Factor Surveillance System has reported that less than 20% of adults get the recommended amount of physical activity every day; moreover, 25% of adults are completely sedentary [56]. This risk is even more significant in the rural population. In fact, Parks and colleagues [57] found that suburban, higher-income residents were more than twice as likely to meet physical activity requirements as rural, lower-income residents. Barriers to getting physical activity (lack of shopping malls, gyms, walking trails, and safe streets) as well as the lack of social support were significant factors, but low income was the common denominator in all inactive groups. Children are always learning and often adopt the behaviors modeled to them. Sedentary caretakers facilitate more television viewing and less activity in children [26]. When school children in a rural Georgia community were studied, 48% were obese or at risk of overweight, and these same children already had an increased incidence of metabolic syndrome, including hypertension and hypercholesterolemia [51]. If no significant intervention to reduce the prevalence of obesity occurs in the lives of these children, it is inevitable that they will develop many of the same cardiovascular complications that are present in their parents.

Special issues related to agriculture

Agricultural pesticides

Case 1: A 9-year-old secretly watched her neighbor crop dusting, and a little spray drifted onto her skin and clothes. A few hours later, she developed a skin rash and vomiting. The pesticide spray included methyl parathion, an organophosphate insecticide.

Case 2: A migrant farm family including five children from 2 to 14 years in age arrived early at a worksite to talk with the farmer. While waiting, the children played in the field and on a utility truck. The family members experienced a variety of symptoms, including rashes, dizziness, shortness of breath, and chest pain, beginning about 6 hours after leaving the field. The field had just been sprayed with the herbicides Upbeat and Betanex, which are generally low in toxicity.

As these cases indicate, children living in rural areas have unique opportunities for accidental exposure to agricultural pesticides. The vast majority of both urban and rural families use pesticides in and around the home to control pests such as roaches, ants, and mice [58]. The main difference is that children who live near agriculture can have low-level exposure to agricultural pesticides [59], including organophosphates, or accidental acute poisoning, in addition to regular exposure to household pesticides and foodborne residues. One exposure route that sometimes is overlooked is carry-home transport of pesticide residues on the shoes and clothing of working parents [60]. A prudent approach for farm workers is to minimize pesticide exposure to themselves and their children by washing hands before eating, removing work shoes and changing clothes before entering the house, and carefully washing contaminated clothes in hot water separate from the clothes of the rest of the family.

Children of migrant farm workers may be at particular risk for pesticide exposure. Youth under age 13 years often accompany parents in the field because of the lack of child care, transportation, or finances. When field workers are paid by piece or weight of product harvested, children working along side their parents or older siblings can help increase the family's earnings. Lack of field sanitation, water for hand washing, and proximity to other workers wearing contaminated clothing increase pesticide exposure. The effect of low-level, chronic exposure to pesticide residues is uncertain. Rural Latino preschool children living near areas where agricultural pesticides are used have demonstrated lower performance on neurobehavioral tests than rural controls not exposed to agriculture [61,62]. Whether these children catch up with their peers in later years or lag behind them permanently is unknown.

Occupational injuries to children doing farm work

Growing up on a farm has advantages for children [63]; however, farm work can be very dangerous because of a wide array of occupational and environmental hazards. On average, about 100 children are killed on farms in the United States each year, and nearly 23,000 are hurt in the process of doing farm work [64,65]. Although the US Federal child-labor laws prohibit children from working in most hazardous occupations, family-owned farms are exempt from child-labor laws [66]. It is common for children who grow up on a farm to be assigned regular tasks in crop and livestock husbandry from an early age [67]. The farm youth work force is comprised of both youth who live on the farm and those who live elsewhere but are hired to do farm work [65]. An estimated 32,800 restricted-activity injuries occurred in youth less than 20 years old who lived, visited, or were hired to work on a farm in 1998. Of these injuries, about 14,600 were related to doing work or chores on the farm [65]. Injuries in working farm children often result from falls/rollovers from tractors, falls from equipment or ladders, and entanglement in power take-off shafts (a rapidly rotating mechanism for transferring power from the engine of the tractor to an ancillary piece of equipment) or other machine components such as augers that may result in amputation or death [68–70].

Agencies such as the National Institute of Occupational Safety and Health and the US Department of Agriculture have sponsored safety programs to help both supervising adults and children gain awareness of work hazards, injury risk, and prevention strategies. Many of these programs are listed in the next section. Unfortunately, knowledge does not always translate into behavior adoption or change. Farms remain a challenging frontier for safety, with many children severely injured or killed every year as a result of activities on farms in the United States.

Summary and resources

The following list highlights facets of the rural environment that were discussed in this article and lists some resources for the clinician to address problems associated with the rural environment.

- Air quality
    Environmental history: for children who have pulmonary disease, consider dust exposure, proximity to CAFOs, farm tasks, and household smoking
    Air quality data: United States Environmental Protection Agency (US EPA)—AirData: Access to Air Pollution Data, http://www.epa.gov/air/data/index.html, or US Department of Agriculture (USDA—Agricultural Air Quality Task Force, http://www.airquality.nrcs.usda.gov/AAQTF/index.html
    Tobacco smoke: Tobacco Information and Prevention Service (TIPS) 4 Youth, http://www.cdc.gov/tobacco/tips4youth.htm; Smoking Cessation, http://www.cancer.org/docroot/home/index.asp; Toll-free counseling: 1-800- ACS-2345
- Water quality
    Environmental history: for children who have gastrointestinal disorders and tooth decay, consider drinking water source and sewage system
    Well water guidance: Drinking Water from Household Wells, EPA, http://www.epa.gov/safewater/privatewells/booklet/index.html
    Septic system risk questionnaire from Purdue, http://www.purdue.edu/dp/envirosoft/septics/src/waste_assess.htm
    Farm*A*Syst: self-administered worksheets and fact sheets pertaining to pollution prevention of wells and other areas, http://www.uwex.edu/farmasyst/index.html
    Recommendations for using fluoride to prevent and control dental caries in the United States, http://www.cdc.gov/mmwr/preview/mmwrhtml/rr5014a1.htm
- Animal safety
    Environmental history: for children who live near livestock or with a hunting family, include anticipatory guidance on animal safety and firearms
    USDA Cooperative State Research, Education, and Extension Service, by state, http://www.csrees.usda.gov/qlinks/partners/state_partners.html
    Lifestock Safety for Kids, a 10-minute video in English and Spanish, order from http://www.swagcenter.org/kids_safety.htm
- Rural motor vehicle safety: encourage seat belts and child safety seats
    All-Terrain Vehicle Safety Fact Sheet from the American Academy of Orthopedic Surgeons, http://orthoinfo.aaos.org/fact/thr_report.cfm?Thread_ID=341&topcategory=Injury%20Prevention

- Rural drowning prevention: convey increased fatality of rural immersion
  National Ag Safety Database, Farm Pond Safety, http://www.cdc.gov/nasd/docs/d001001-d001100/d001009/d001009.html
- Rural lifestyle and obesity: recommend walking, biking, physical education in school, avoidance of sweetened drinks
  Active Living by Design, see rural programs in Isanti County, MN and Upper Valley, NH/VT, http://www.activelivingbydesign.org/index.php?id=6
- Pesticide safety: recommend minimizing farm children's exposure by creating a safe play area
  Safe play booklet from the National Children's Center for Rural and Agricultural Health and Safety, http://www.marshfieldclinic.org/nfmc/Pages/Proxy.aspx?Content=MCRF-Centers-NFMC-keyprojects-booklet-safeplay-v2.1.pdf;
  For acute poisonings, contact the Poison Control Center, http://www.aapcc.org/; consultation line: 1-800-222-1222
  For information about long-term exposures, contact the local Pediatric Environmental Health Specialty Unit. Contact information is available at http://www.aoec.org/PEHSU.htm or 1-888-347-AOEC (2632)
  For other toxicity questions, contact the National Pesticide Information Center, http://npic.orst.edu/index.html; Information line: 1-800-858-7378
- Youth working in agriculture: Raise awareness of safety concerns
  Occupational Safety and Health Act Guide to Teen Workers, including Youth in Agriculture e-tool, http://www.osha.gov/SLTC/teenworkers/index.html
  Farm Safety for Kids, http://www.fs4jk.org/
  North American Guidelines for Children's Agricultural Tasks, http://www.nagcat.org/nagcat/pages/default.aspx
- Overview of Rural and Farm Hazards
  National Library of Medicine, Tox Town, Farm Scene, http://toxtown.nlm.nih.gov/
  National Ag Safety Database, http://www.cdc.gov/nasd/

Acknowledgment

The authors thank Jeff Levin, MD, Victoria Butler, MD, Tom Cherry, MD, Larry Lowry, PhD, and Torey Nalbone, PhD, for their help in reviewing this manuscript.

References

[1] Goldsmith HF, Puskin DS, Stilles DJ. Improving the operational definition of "Rural Areas" for federal programs. Rockville, MD: Department of Health and Human Services,

Federal Office of Rural Health Policy; 1993. Available at: http://ruralhealth.hrsa.gov/pub/
Goldsmith.htm. Accessed January 25, 2007.

[2] Ricketts T. Rural health in the United States. New York: Oxford University Press; 1999.

[3] Gracey M. Child health implications of worldwide urbanization. Rev Environ Health 2003;
18(1):51–63.

[4] Rogers CC. Rural children at a glance. Washington, DC: U.S. Department of Agriculture, USDA Economic Research Service; 2005. Available at: http://www.ers.usda.gov/
publications/EIB1/EIB1.pdf. Accessed January 25, 2007.

[5] Glasgow N, Morton LW, Johnson NE, editors. Critical issues in rural health. Ames (IA):
Blackwell Publishing; 2004.

[6] Mather M. Rural kids lagging in health, education. Rural Families Data Center. July 2004.
Available at: http://www.prb.org/rfdcenter/ruralkidsllagginginhlth.htm. Accessed January
24, 2007.

[7] Grunbaum J. Youth risk behavior surveillance, 2001. MMWR CDC Surveill Summ 2002;
51(SS-4):1–64.

[8] Grunbaum J, Kann L, Kinchen S, et al. Youth risk behavior surveillance—United States
2003. MMWR CDC Surveill Summ 2004;53(SS-02):1–96.

[9] Campbell-Grossman C, Hudson DB, Fleck MO. Chewing tobacco use: perceptions and
knowledge in rural adolescent youths. Issues Compr Pediatr Nurs 2003;26(1):13–21.

[10] Lineberry TW, Bostwick JM. Methamphetamine abuse: a perfect storm of complications.
Mayo Clin Proc 2006;81(1):77–84.

[11] Mittlestadt M. Illegal immigrants make up 5% of workforce, study finds. Dallas Morning
News. March 8, 2006. Available at: http://www.dallasnews.com/s/dws/bus/stories/DN-
pewstudy_08bus.ART0.State.Edition2.8496.html. Accessed January 25, 2007.

[12] Kline J, Schwartz D. Agricultural dust-induced lung disease. In: Rom WN, editor. Environmental and occupational medicine. 3rd edition. Philadelphia: Lippincott-Raven Publishers;
1998. p. 565–71.

[13] Anonymous. Respiratory health hazards in agriculture. Am J Respir Crit Care Med 1998;
158(5 Pt 2):S1–76.

[14] Meggs J, Langley R, James P. Farm toxicology. In: Goldfrank LR, editor. Goldfrank's toxicologic emergencies. 7th edition. New York: McGraw-Hill; 2002. p. 1690–8.

[15] Stevens S, Colwell B, Hutchison S. Tobacco use in rural areas: a literature review. Rural
healthy people 2010: a companion document to healthy people 2010. vol 2. College Station
(TX): The Texas A&M University System Health Science Center, School of Rural Public
Health, Southwest Rural Health Research Center; 2003.

[16] Iverson L, Hannaford P, Price D, et al. Is living in a rural area good for your respiratory
health? Results from a cross-sectional study in Scotland. Chest 2005;128(4):2059–67.

[17] Adler A, Tager I, Quintero DR. Decreased prevalence of asthma among farm-reared
children compared with those who are rural but not farm-reared. J Allergy Clin Immunol
2005;115(1):67–73.

[18] Higgins PS, Wakefield D, Cloutier MM. Risk factors for asthma and asthma severity in
nonurban children in Connecticut. Chest 2005;128(6):3846–53.

[19] von Mutius E. Influences in allergy: epidemiology and the environment. J Allergy Clin
Immunol 2004;113(3):373–9 [quiz: 380].

[20] Riedler J, Braun-Fahrlander C, Eder W, et al. Exposure to farming in early life and development of asthma and allergy: a cross-sectional survey. Lancet 2001;358(9288):1129–33.

[21] EPA. Water on tap: what you need to know (4601). Office of Water Quality. EPA-816-
K-003–07. Environmental Protection Agency; 2003.

[22] EPA. Drinking water from household wells. EPA 816-K-02–003. Environmental Protection
Agency; 2002.

[23] Borchardt MA, Chyou PH, DeVries EO, et al. Septic system density and infectious diarrhea
in a defined population of children. Environ Health Perspect 2003;111(5):742–8.

[24] EPA. National management measures for the control of nonpoint pollution from agriculture. EPA-841-B-03-004; 2003.

[25] EPA. National Pollutant Discharge Elimination System (NPDES). Animal feeding operations: frequently asked questions. Available at: http://cfpub.epa.gov/npdes/faqs.cfm. Accessed January 24, 2007.

[26] Polley DC, Spicer MT, Knight AP, et al. Intrafamilial correlates of overweight and obesity in African-American and Native-American grandparents, parents, and children in rural Oklahoma. J Am Diet Assoc 2005;105(2):262–5.

[27] Barnes GP, Parker WA, Lyon TC Jr, et al. Ethnicity, location, age, and fluoridation factors in baby bottle tooth decay and caries prevalence of Head Start children. Public Health Rep 1992;107(2):167–73.

[28] CDC. Injuries among youth on farms in the United States, 1998. DHHS (NIOSH) Publication No. 2001-154. 2001.

[29] Norwood S, McAuley C, Vallina VL, et al. Mechanisms and patterns of injuries related to large animals. Journal of Trauma-Injury Infection & Critical Care 2000;48(4):740–4.

[30] Cyr D, Johnson S. Child safety around animals. Maine Farm Safety Fact Sheet 2002. Available at: http://www.cdc.gov/NASD/docs/d000701-d000800/d000796/d000796.html. Accessed January 24, 2007.

[31] CDC. Interim guidance for protection of persons involved in U.S. avian influenza outbreak disease control and eradication activities. Atlanta, GA: Department of Health and Human Services; 2004. Available at: http://cdc.gov/flu/avian/professional/pdf/protectionguid.pdf. Accessed January 25, 2007.

[32] Pickett W, Brison RJ, Berg RL, et al. Pediatric farm injuries involving non-working children injured by a farm work hazard: five priorities for primary prevention. Inj Prev 2005;11(1): 6–11.

[33] Eber GB, Annest JL, Mercy JA, et al. Nonfatal and fatal firearm-related injuries among children aged 14 years and younger: United States, 1993-2000. Pediatrics 2004;113(6):1686–92.

[34] Rausch TK, Sanddal ND, Sanddal TL, et al. Changing epidemiology of injury-related pediatric mortality in a rural state: implications for injury control. Pediatr Emerg Care 1998; 14(6):388–92.

[35] Sinauer N, Annest JL, Mercy JA. Unintentional, nonfatal firearm-related injuries. A preventable public health burden. JAMA 1996;275(22):1740–3.

[36] Connor SM, Wesolowski KL. "They're too smart for that": predicting what children would do in the presence of guns. Pediatrics 2003;111(2):E109–14.

[37] Muellerman RL, Walker RA, Edney JA. Motor vehicle deaths: a rural epidemic. Journal of Trauma-Injury Infection & Critical Care 1993;35(5):717–9.

[38] Clark DE, Cushing BM. Rural and urban traffic fatalities, vehicle miles, and population density. Accid Anal Prev 2004;36(6):967–72.

[39] Zwerling C, Peek-Asa C, Whitten PS, et al. Fatal motor vehicle crashes in rural and urban areas: decomposing rates into contributing factors. Inj Prev 2005;11(1):24–8.

[40] Schootman M, Fuortes LJ, Zwerling C, et al. Safety behavior among Iowa junior high and high school students. Am J Public Health 1993;83(11):1628–30.

[41] King WD, Nichols MH, Hardwick WE, et al. Urban/rural differences in child passenger deaths. Pediatr Emerg Care 1994;10(1):34–6.

[42] Rogers FB, Shackford SR, Hoyt DB, et al. Trauma deaths in a mature urban vs rural trauma system. A comparison. Arch Surg 1997;132(4):376–81.

[43] Anonymous. All-terrain vehicle injury prevention: two-, three-, and four-wheeled unlicensed motor vehicles [see comment]. Pediatrics 2000;105(6):1352–4.

[44] Killingsworth JB, Tilford JM, Parker JG, et al. National hospitalization impact of pediatric all-terrain vehicle injuries. Pediatrics 2005;115(3):e316–21.

[45] Cvijanovich NZ, Cook LJ, Mann NC, et al. A population-based assessment of pediatric all-terrain vehicle injuries. Pediatrics 2001;108(3):631–5.

[46] Goldcamp M, Hendricks KJ, Myers JR. Farm fatalities to youth 1995-2000: a comparison by age groups. J Safety Res 2004;35(2):151–7.
[47] Adekoya N. Trends in childhood drowning on U.S. farms, 1986-1997. J Rural Health 2003; 19(1):11–4.
[48] Bugeja L, Franklin R. Drowning deaths of zero- to five-year-old children in Victorian dams, 1989-2001. Aust J Rural Health 2005;13(5):300–8.
[49] Nixon J, Pearn J, Wilkey I, et al. Fifteen years of child drowning—a 1967-1981 analysis of all fatal cases from the Brisbane Drowning Study and an 11 year study of consecutive near-drowning cases. Accid Anal Prev 1986;18(3):199–203.
[50] O'Flaherty JE, Pirie PL. Prevention of pediatric drowning and near-drowning: a survey of members of the American Academy of Pediatrics. Pediatrics 1997;99(2):169–74.
[51] Davis CL, Flickinger B, Moore D, et al. Prevalence of cardiovascular risk factors in school-children in a rural Georgia community. Am J Med Sci 2005;330(2):53–9.
[52] Davy BM, Harrell K, Stewart J, et al. Body weight status, dietary habits, and physical activity levels of middle school-aged children in rural Mississippi. South Med J 2004;97(6):571–7.
[53] Demerath E, Muratova V, Spangler E, et al. School-based obesity screening in rural Appalachia. Prev Med 2003;37(6 Pt 1):553–60.
[54] Liebman M, Pelican S, Moore SA, et al. Dietary intake, eating behavior, and physical activity-related determinants of high body mass index in rural communities in Wyoming, Montana, and Idaho. Int J Obes Relat Metab Disord 2003;27(6):684–92.
[55] McMurray RG, Harrell JS, Bangdiwala SI, et al. Cardiovascular disease risk factors and obesity of rural and urban elementary school children. J Rural Health 1999;15(4):365–74.
[56] CDC. Surveillance for certain health behaviors among states and selected local areas—behavioral risk factor surveillance system, United States, 2003. MMWR Surveill Summ 2005;54(SS08):1–116.
[57] Parks SE, Housemann RA, Brownson RC. Differential correlates of physical activity in urban and rural adults of various socioeconomic backgrounds in the United States. J Epidemiol Community Health 2003;57(1):29–35.
[58] Adgate JL, Kukowski A, Stroebel C, et al. Pesticide storage and use patterns in Minnesota households with children. J Expo Anal Environ Epidemiol 2000;10(2):159–67.
[59] Freeman NC, Shalat SL, Black K, et al. Seasonal pesticide use in a rural community on the US/Mexico border. J Expo Anal Environ Epidemiol 2004;14(6):473–8.
[60] Lambert WE, Lasarev M, Muniz J, et al. Variation in organophosphate pesticide metabolites in urine of children living in agricultural communities. Environ Health Perspect 2005;113(4):504–8.
[61] Guillette EA, Meza MM, Aquilar MG, et al. An anthropological approach to the evaluation of preschool children exposed to pesticides in Mexico. Environ Health Perspect 1998;106(6):347–53.
[62] Rohlman DS, Arcury TA, Quandt SA, et al. Neurobehavioral performance in preschool children from agricultural and non-agricultural communities in Oregon and North Carolina. Neurotoxicology 2005;26(4):589–98.
[63] Larson NC, Dearmont M. Strengths of farming communities in fostering resilience in children. Child Welfare 2002;81(5):821–35.
[64] Adekoya N, Pratt S. Fatal unintentional farm injuries among persons less than 20 years of age: geographic profiles. DHHS/NIOSH Publication No. 2001-131. 2001.
[65] Myers JR, Hendricks KJ. Injuries among youth on farms in the United States, 1998. DHHS/NIOSH publication No. 2001-154. 2001.
[66] Perry MJ. Children's agricultural health: traumatic injuries and hazardous inorganic exposures. J Rural Health 2003;19(3):269–78.
[67] Marlenga B, Pickett W, Berg RL. Agricultural work activities reported for children and youth on 498 North American farms. J Agric Saf Health 2001;7(4):241–52.
[68] Hard D, Myers J, Snyder K, et al. Young workers at risk when working in agricultural production. Am J Ind Med 1999;(Suppl 1):31–3.

[69] Gerberich SG, Gibson RW, French LR, et al. Injuries among children and youth in farm households: Regional Rural Injury Study—I. Inj Prev 2001;7(2):117–22.
[70] Rivara FP. Fatal and non-fatal farm injuries to children and adolescents in the United States, 1990-3 [see comment]. Inj Prev 1997;3(3):190–4.

PEDIATRIC CLINICS

OF NORTH AMERICA

Pediatr Clin N Am
54 (2007) 135–153

The Use of the Internet for Children's Health and the Environment

Jerome A. Paulson, MD, FAAP[a,b,c,*],
Stacey J. Arnesen, MS[d]

[a]George Washington University School of Medicine and Health Sciences, 2300 I Street NW,
Washington, DC 20037, USA
[b]George Washington University School of Public Health and Health Services,
2300 I Street NW, Washington, DC 20037, USA
[c]Mid-Atlantic Center for Children's Health and the Environment,
2300 M Street NW, #203, Washington, DC 20052, USA
[d]Specialized Information Services, National Library of Medicine,
6707 Democracy Blvd., Bethesda, MD 20892, USA

The use of the Internet for all medical purposes has grown tremendously in the last several decades [1–4]. Among professionals the Internet can be used as a means of communication (ie, e-mail) and, as emphasized in this article, as a means of information retrieval.

The Internet, also known as the World Wide Web, is particularly useful for retrieving information related to children's environmental health. Many international agencies, many governmental agencies in the United States, Canada, and elsewhere, and many nongovernmental organizations (NGOs) have created websites specifically to disseminate environmental health information. In fact, some environmental health information, for example, some of the toxicology and other databases on the National Library of Medicine (NLM) Website (http://tox.nlm.nih.gov) or NGO Websites such as Scorecard (http://scorecard.org/), are available only on the Internet.

Bonus material pertaining to this article is available online at www.pediatric.theclinics.com. See notation within this article for details.

This work was supported through a grant from the Association of Occupational & Environmental Clinics under a cooperative agreement with the Agency for Toxic Substances and Disease Registry and the US Environmental Protection Agency.

* Corresponding author. Mid-Atlantic Center for Children's Health & the Environment, 2300 M Street, NW, #203, Washington, DC 20052.

E-mail address: jpaulson@cnmc.org (J.A. Paulson).

doi:10.1016/j.pcl.2006.11.011

Obtaining information about children's environmental health on the Internet

Numerous government agencies, organizations, and medical associations have developed Web-based resources and/or databases related to environmental health and toxicology. This section highlights the NLM resources and reviews several other government agencies and organizations. Information about additional environmental health and toxicology resources can be found on the NLM's Toxicology Web Links web page (http://sis.nlm.nih.gov/enviro/toxweblinks.html).

Because of the reliability of information on these sites, their ease of use, and the ability to reach so many databases simultaneously if needed, these sites should be the first accessed when searching for information about children's health and the environment.

National Library of Medicine's Toxicology and Environmental Health Information Program

Since the late 1960s, the NLM's Toxicology and Environmental Health Information Program has developed and made accessible databases and other resources for the scientific community and, more recently, for the public. The NLM's Environmental Health and Toxicology Portal (Fig. 1) contains links to an extensive collection of databases and other Web-based resources covering many environmental health and toxicology topics. These resources include bibliographic databases, online toxicology handbooks, a chemical and drug dictionary, directories, webliogrpahies (bibliographies of Web links or a list of links), and tutorials in toxicology.

One of NLM's major resources is TOXNET (http://toxnet.nlm.nih.gov), a collection of databases (Box 1).

The databases listed in Box 1 are primarily oriented toward health professionals and scientists. Following a government-wide effort to create and provide health information to the general public, the NLM recently created several new resources designed for a wider audience (Box 2).

As a portal for environmental health information, the NLH's Toxicology and Environmental Health Information Program website (http://tox.nlm.nih.gov) contains other useful resources (Box 3).

Other websites of interest for children's environmental health

Agencies of the United States government

The US Environmental Protection Agency (EPA) (www.epa.gov) is the primary federal agency responsible for protecting human health and the environment. The EPA has the authority to promulgate regulations to improve the environment and protect human health. The EPA has a number of program offices (eg, air, water, research and development), regional offices, and laboratories. The Office of Children's Health Protection

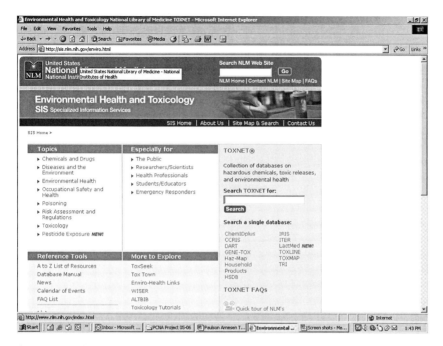

Fig. 1. Screen shot of the National Library of Medicine Environmental Health and Toxicology Portal.

(http://yosemite.epa.gov/ochp/ochpweb.nsf/homepage) is part of the Office of the EPA Administrator. The Office of Children's Health Protection and the other program offices maintain an extensive set of web pages. Many are accessible from a menu on the EPA home page (www.epa.gov), where one can click, for example, on lead (http://www.epa.gov/lead/), or water (http://www.epa.gov/ebtpages/water.html), or acid rain (http://www.epa.gov/airmarkets/arp/), or mold (http://www.epa.gov/mold/moldresources.html). Along the left side of the EPA home page is a menu where one can click on Information Sources (http://www.epa.gov/epahome/resource.htm) to access an extensive catalogue of information and materials available from the EPA. Within that page, one can click on Databases and Software (http://www.epa.gov/epahome/Data.html) to find a list of online and downloadable tools to access environmental data from the EPA. Some materials of specific interest might include Envirofacts (http://www.epa.gov/enviro/), a national information system that provides a single point of access to data extracted from seven major EPA databases, and Window To My Environment (http://www.epa.gov/enviro/wme/), a program that uses interactive maps and tools to answer popular questions about local environmental conditions affecting air, land, and water.

The Agency for Toxic Substances and Disease Registry (ATSDR) (http://www.atsdr.cdc.gov/), a part of the US Department of Health and Human

Box 1. Databases in TOXNET
(Available at: http://toxnet.nlm.nih.gov/)

- ChemIDplus: dictionary of nearly 400,000 chemicals (names, synonyms, structures); includes links to chemical information from NLM resources and other resources
- Hazardous Substances Data Bank (HSDB): comprehensive peer-reviewed toxicologic data on approximately 4800 chemicals; contains excerpts from the published literature and covers human health effects, emergency medical treatment, animal toxicity studies, environmental fate and exposure, standards and regulations, chemical safety and handling, chemical and physical properties, and manufacturing and use information
- TOXLINE: contains more than 3 million references from MEDLINE/PubMed (TOXLINE Core) and other toxicology literature, including research in progress and meeting abstracts (TOXLINE Special)
- Chemical Carcinogenesis Research Information System (CCRIS): a National Cancer Institute database on the testing of more than 8000 chemicals for carcinogenicity, mutagenicity, tumor promotion, and tumor inhibition
- Developmental and Reproductive Toxicology (DART): contains more than 225,000 references to the teratology, developmental, and reproductive toxicology literature from 1980 to the present
- GENETOX: Peer-reviewed mutagenicity test data from Environmental Protection Agency (EPA)
- Integrated Risk Information System (IRIS) hazard identification and dose-response assessment data on more than 500 chemicals
- International Toxicity Estimates of Risk (ITER) chemical risk data from resources world wide
- LactMed: peer-reviewed and fully referenced database of drugs to which breastfeeding mothers may be exposed. Includes maternal and infant levels of drugs, possible effects on breastfed infants and on lactation, and alternate drugs to consider.
- Toxics Release Inventory (TRI): an EPA database of annual reports on the environmental release of more than 600 chemicals by industrial facilities in the United States
- Haz-Map: an occupational health database designed for health and safety professionals and for consumers seeking

information about the health effects of exposure to chemicals and biologicals at work
- Household Products Database: This database links many consumer products to health effects information from Material Safety Data Sheets (MSDS) provided by the manufacturers.
- TOXMAP: a geographic information system displaying interactive maps of TRI, Superfund, and other health and demographic data; provides links to additional information on the toxic chemicals

Services and closely linked to the National Center for Environmental Health of the Centers for Disease Control (CDC), has a number of responsibilities that include gathering and maintaining information concerning the effect of hazardous substances in the environment on public health. It publishes a series of documents known as "Toxicological Profiles" containing detailed information on several hundred chemicals (http://www.atsdr.cdc.gov/toxpro2.html). All the Toxicological Profiles contain a section specifically on the health hazards of the substance to children. The ATSDR also creates easy-to-read excerpts of these profiles called "ToxFAQs" (http://www.atsdr.cdc.gov/toxfaq.html), which can be very useful for providing information to patients and at public meetings.

Box 2. National Library of Medicine databases targeted for the general public

- Tox Town (http://toxtown.nlm.nih.gov): an interactive guide to potentially toxic substances and environmental health issues in everyday places. Several scenes, including a town, city, farm, and the US-Mexico border are available for exploration.
- Household products (http://householdproducts.nlm.nih.gov): a database of more than 6000 household products, their ingredients, and potential health effects; information is derived from product labels and Material Safety Data Sheets (MSDS).
- MedlinePlus (http://medlineplus.gov): links to authoritative health information on more than 700 health topics, including more than 30 environmental health and toxicology topics (http://ww.nlm.nih.gov/medlineplus/poisoningtoxicologyenvironmentalhealth.html); also contains interactive tutorials, drug information, a medical dictionary and encyclopedia, and directories of health professionals and organizations in the United States; also available in Spanish

---

**Box 3. Resources available at the NLH's Toxicology
and Environmental Health Information Program Web site
(http://tox.nlm.nih.gov)**

- Toxicology Tutorials (Tox Tutor): a series of three tutorials on
  the basic principles of toxicology, toxicokinetics, and cellular
  toxicology. The NLM and the U.S. Society of Toxicology
  currently are updating and expanding these tutorials.
- Enviro-Health Links (http://sis.nlm.nih.gov/enviro/
  envirohealthlinks.html): summaries and "lists of links" or
  webliographies on current topics of interest in toxicology and
  environmental health including
  o Children's environmental health (http://phpartners.org/cehir/
    sampler.html)
  o Arctic health
  o Agents of chemical and biologic warfare
  o Arsenic
  o Indoor and outdoor air pollution
  o Pesticide exposure
  o West Nile virus
  o Toxicogenomics
  o General toxicology
  o Education and careers in toxicology and environmental
    health
- Tox-Enviro Listserv: an announcements-only listserv to keep
  up-to-date with new environmental health and toxicology
  resources from NLM. Join by registering at http://
  sis.nlm.nih.gov/enviro/envirolistserv.html.
- DIRLINE (http://dirline.nlm.nih.gov): a directory
  of health-related organizations including several hundred
  environmental health and children's health resources

In addition, the ATSDR has developed two continuing education case studies related to children's environmental health: Pediatric Environmental Health (http://www.atsdr.cdc.gov/HEC/CSEM/pediatric/index.html) and Environmental Triggers of Asthma (http://www.atsdr.cdc.gov/HEC/CSEM/asthma/index.html). These case studies are part of a series of self-instructional publications designed to increase the primary care provider's knowledge of hazardous substances in the environment and to aid in the evaluation of potentially exposed patients. Continuing medical education, continuing nursing education, and continuing education credits are provided.

The National Center for Environmental Health (http://www.cdc.gov/nceh/) of the CDC provides public health surveillance and applied research related to environmental health hazards. Its website provides information on air pollution (http://www.cdc.gov/nceh/airpollution/), asthma (http://www.cdc.gov/asthma/default.htm), lead exposure (http://www.cdc.gov/nceh/lead/lead.htm), and a number of other topics. One of the most important recent undertakings of the National Center for Environmental Health related to children's health is the National Exposures Report. This report, based on information collected from a representative sample of the noninstitutionalized United States population, measures chemicals or their metabolites in blood, urine, or other biologic materials. The most recent report of biomonitoring described the presence of 148 chemicals in people of all ages is the United States (http://www.cdc.gov/exposurereport/).

Other resources

A number of organizations have children's environmental health as their primary or significant focus. The Children's Environmental Health Network (CHEN) (http://www.cehn.org) is one of the major organizations providing information to health care professionals and the public. CEHN is a national, multidisciplinary organization dedicated to protecting the fetus and the child from environmental hazards and to promoting a healthy environment. Its website provides an overview of children's environmental health issues, a training manual on pediatric environmental health, and a resource guide of related programs, projects, and organizations. The CEHN also sponsors listservs for the exchange of ideas related to children's environmental health.

Another organization, the Children's Health Environmental Coalition (http://www.checnet.org), works to educate the public, specifically parents and caregivers, about environmental toxins that affect children's health. Although the information is geared toward consumers, the resources also are useful for health professionals. The Children's Health Environmental Coalition has developed an interactive resource, Health*e*House, for information about environmental health risks children face at home. All of the information is reviewed by toxicologists and endorsed by the Children's Health Environmental Coalition Science Advisory Committee.

The American Academy of Pediatrics website (http://www.aap.org/healthtopics/environmentalhealth.cfm) contains several articles on various children's environmental health topics including lead and mercury poisoning, air pollution, and terrorism. The American Academy of Pediatrics also published the second edition of *Pediatric Environmental Health* in 2003.

International organizations also are working to reduce environmental health risks to children. For example, the World Health Organization sponsors a Task Force for the Protection of Children's Environmental Health (http://www.who.int/ceh/en/). The mission is to prevent disease and disability in children associated with chemical and physical threats and biologic risks in the environment. The website contains basic information on children's environmental health issues and descriptions on ongoing projects and national profiles.

There are dozens of websites with information about children's health and the environment. The web-based version of this article contains a table listing many of those resources.

Other means of finding information on the Internet

The Internet is so useful because it allows anyone with access to a computer with web browser software and a connection to the Internet to look at information in multiple formats: text, photographic, and other graphic formats, tables, sound, and video. An advantage unique to the Internet is easy and rapid linking from one document to another.

One of the challenges to the use of the Internet is finding the information that one wants in a timely fashion. There are millions of websites and billions of individual's web pages, and there are several different approaches to finding information [5].

Browsing

One can identify a particular website that is useful. Many sites have identified links (ie, the addresses [URLs], of other similar websites). One can follow those links electronically to the other sites. This process is known as browsing. Although it can be helpful at times, it often is inefficient, and the links may be to a very narrow range of sites.

Searching

It is more desirable to use some methodology to search actively for and identify websites. One can use web search engines, web directories, or web indexes. Most individuals will be familiar with one or more if the better-known search engines: Google (www.google.com), Yahoo! (www.yahoo.com,), and LookSmart (www.looksmart.com). Some search engines have been created to search other search engines; these include Dogpile (www.dogpile.com) and Search.com (www.search.com). All search engines have a box in which to enter search terms. In determining which search engine to use, one should look for advanced search capabilities, such as the ability to combine words or to search for exact phrases, and consider the ease of use of the search site.

Other search methods

Many websites have an internal search system. Often, there is a box labeled "search," in which one may enter a term and look for information within the site itself. For example, the EPA website (www.epa.gov) has a search box in the center of the page and a link to a page that allows one to do more advanced searching. Also on the EPA home page is an example of a directory—a list of EPA's major topics—that allows rapid access to the appropriate pages within the EPA website. Many other Web sites, such as the Centers for Disease Control and Prevention (www.cdc.gov) or the Natural Resources Defense Council (www.nrdc.org), also have internal search engines and directories.

Databases

Databases can provide quick and efficient access to specific detailed information on a topic. An earlier section provided detailed information about some of the databases maintained by the NLM and other organizations. In some instances, it may be useful to search more than one database for information [6].

Evaluating websites

The Internet's ease of access to a myriad of information is also one of its pitfalls. Anyone with a modicum of skill can post information on the Internet. Unlike most print media or radio or television, there are no editors, no fact checkers, and no other overall means of control. One way to conceive of the Internet is as a huge bookshelf housing books created by individuals with various levels of skills and with various points of view. A book's presence on the shelf does not mean that it is a good or accurate book.

Because the use of the Internet is very much a caveat emptor situation, one must scrutinize a website and decide on the reliability of the information that it contains. The URL gives some information about the origin of the website. For example, the last three letters of the URL constitute the domain name. Most people are familiar with the phrase, "dot com," which technically means a website created by a commercial enterprise. The domain name ".org" usually means a website created by a nonprofit organization, and the domain name ".gov" indicates a website created by a nonmilitary US governmental (federal or state) entity. By looking at the domain name, one can begin to make a judgment about the material on the website (Table 1).

Several organizations have developed criteria for evaluating a website. With funding from the US Agency for Health Care Policy and Research,

Table 1
Domain names

Domain Name	Type of Site
.com	commercial site
.net	commercial site
.gov	US government site
.org	nonprofit site
.edu	higher education organization site
.mil	US military site
.biz	commercial site
.int	international site
country code	two-letter code indicating the country (eg, .br for Brazil and .ca for Canada)

the Health Summit Working Group published *Criteria for Assessing the Quality of Health Information on the Internet - Policy Paper* (Box 4) [7]. Although this document was created to provide suggestions for the evaluation of consumer-oriented website, the criteria also are useful for professionals, particularly in an area such as environmental health, in which evidence-based data are limited and claims may outstrip factual support. The NLM has created an online tutorial on evaluating health information on the Internet. It is targeted more towards consumers than towards professionals but could be of use to all. It is available at http://www.nlm.nih.gov/medlineplus/webeval/webeval.html.

Looking at a website, one should be able to determine who created the content of the site, that is, the author of the site, the affiliation of the creator, and a means for contacting the creator. The purpose of the site—to provide information or to sell a product—should be stated clearly. One of the challenges is gauging the accuracy of the information contained in the site. An academic medical center or a US government entity such as the NLM has more credibility and is more likely to provide accurate information about environmental health than Sam the barber. The site should reveal whether the information posted was subject to any system of review. Information on websites should be dated. In a field that changes as rapidly as environmental health, it is important to know if information is outdated. One should be able to identify the source of financial support for a Web site. Just because a website has a commercial sponsor does not make the information invalid, any more than the fact that a website has an academic

---

Box 4. Criteria for evaluating health information found on the Internet

- Credibility: includes the source, currency, relevance/utility, and editorial review process for the information
- Content: must be accurate and complete, and an appropriate disclaimer provided
- Disclosure: includes informing the user of the purpose of the site, as well as any profiling or collection of information associated with using the site
- Links: evaluated according to selection, architecture, content, and back linkages
- Design: encompasses accessibility, logical organization (navigability), and internal search capability
- Interactivity: includes feedback mechanisms and means for exchange of information among users
- Caveats: clarification of whether site function is to market products and services or is a primary information content provider

sponsor or a governmental sponsor makes the information valid. By disclosing information about sponsorship, the creator of the website allows the user to factor that information into an assessment.

The freedom to post material on the Internet has been expanding. In the past, one needed to know certain arcane "languages" such as hypertext markup language (html) to create a web page. Now there are very simple means of creating and modifying web pages. Another new trend is the creation of "wiki" websites. In the past a website could be modified only by its creator or by a hacker. The "wiki" system allows much easier creation of Web sites and also allows anyone to modify the site (usually with a record of the changes). An example of the use of the "wiki" system is the Wikipedia, "the free encyclopedia that anyone can edit" (http://en.wikipedia.org/wiki/Main_Page). The fact that anyone can edit material on "wiki" sites means that the contents must be viewed with great caution.

The Internet frequently has been used to perpetrate outright hoaxes and frauds. If an environmental health claim on the Internet looks too good to be true, it probably is. This problem has been so extensive that the CDC maintains a web page specific to hoaxes that invoke the CDC's name in an attempt to look credible (http://www.cdc.gov/hoax_rumors.htm). Another site that provides information about possible hoaxes and frauds is the Hoaxbusters website maintained by the Computer Incident Advisory Capability of the US Department of Energy (http://hoaxbusters.ciac.org/).

Specific search tools and databases

Table 2 contains a list of key Web sites mentioned in this article. It is not the purpose of this article to promote one commercial search tool over any other.

Google (www.google.com) is one of the most widely used search tools and is considered by some to be one of the better search tools [8]. One component of Google, called "Google US Government" (http://www.google.com/ig/usgov) is relatively unknown but is very useful to individuals looking for information about children's environmental health or other information that may have been developed by a governmental agency. This portion of Google preferentially searches federal and state Web sites in the United States for information. For example, if one were to search for "mercury" in the regular Google website (Fig. 2), the EPA web page on mercury is the seventh item recovered, and one must click through to the third page of results before finding other environmental health information. The same search at Google US Government gives four links related to mercury and environmental health on the first page of results and others on subsequent pages (Fig. 3). All the material in federal Web site has been vetted, making it a good place to start a search. Material in state-sponsored web pages will provide state-specific data and materials, such as brochures, that have been developed for community use.

Table 2
Key Web sites mentioned in the article

Name	Description	Location and Contact
Agency for Toxic Substances and Disease Registry (ATSDR)	ATSDR's highest priority is to protect America's health from toxic exposures.	http://www.atsdr.cdc.gov/
ATSDR Child Health Initiative	Provides summaries of ATSDR child health programs, such as the Pediatric Environmental Health Specialty Units (PEHSUs) as well as links to Toxicology Profiles and Public Health Assessments	http://www.atsdr.cdc.gov/child/
ATSDR Toxicological Profiles	Provides detailed information on individual hazardous chemicals. All profiles include a section on children.	http://www.atsdr.cdc.gov/toxpro2.html
National Center for Environmental Health (NCEH)	Provides national leadership, through science and service, to promote health and quality of life by preventing or controlling those diseases, birth defects, disabilities, or deaths that result from interactions between people and their environment.	http://www.cdc.gov/nceh/
NCEH Asthma Program	—	http://www.cdc.gov/asthma/default.htm
NCEH Lead Poisoning Prevention Program	—	http://www.cdc.gov/nceh/lead/lead.htm
NCEH Human Exposure Report	Reports on the concentrations of chemicals measured in human bodies.	http://www.cdc.gov/exposurereport/
CDC information on hoaxes & rumors	—	http://www.cdc.gov/hoax_rumors.htm
US Environmental Protection Agency (EPA)	—	http://www.epa.gov
EPA Office of Children's Health Protection	The focus within EPA for all issues related to children's health	http://www.epa.gov/children http://yosemite.epa.gov/ochp/ochpweb.nsf/ homepage
EPA Office of Pesticide Programs	The EPA licenses or registers pesticides for use in strict accordance with label directions, based on review of scientific studies on the pesticide to determine that it will not pose unreasonable	http://www.epa.gov/pesticides

EPA Office of Air and Radiation	risks to human health or the environment. For pesticides used on food, EPA sets limits on how much of a pesticide residue may remain in or on foods. EPA also sets standards to protect workers who may be exposed to pesticides on the job.	http://www.epa.gov/oar/ Indoor air web page: http://www.epa.gov/iaq Tools for Schools Program: http://www.epa.gov/iaq/schools/index.html Air Now (ground level ozone): http://www.epa.gov/airnow/
	—	
EPA Endocrine Disruptor Screening Program	The Endocrine Disruptor Screening Program focuses on providing methods and procedures to detect and characterize endocrine activity of pesticides, commercial chemicals, and environmental contaminants.	http://www.epa.gov/scipoly/oscpendo/
EPA Children's Environmental Health Research Initiative	Federal research programs devoted exclusively to children's environmental health and disease prevention	http://cfpub.epa.gov/ncer_abstracts/index.cfm/fuseaction/outlinks.centers
EPA Children's Environmental Health Resource, Toxicity and Exposure Assessment for Children's Health (TEACH)	Searchable database children's environmental health risk from chemical exposure	http://www.epa.gov/teach/
EPA Office of Emergency Management	—	http://www.epa.gov/ceppo/
EPA Office of Water	—	http://www.epa.gov/water/index.html Drinking Water Advisories http://www.epa.gov/waterscience/criteria/drinking/ Fish Consumption Advisories http://www.epa.gov/ost/fish/

(continued on next page)

Table 2 (*continued*)

Name	Description	Location and Contact
EPA Office of Pollution Prevention & Toxics	Administers the Toxic Substances Control Act (TSCA) and the Pollution Prevention Act of 1990. Manages the Chemical Right-to-Know Initiative and the New and Existing Chemicals programs; the Design for the Environment (DFE), Green Chemistry, and Environmentally Preferable Products (EPP) programs; and the Lead, Asbestos, and Polychlorinated Biphenyls (PCBs) programs.	http://www.epa.gov/opptintr/index.html
EPA Healthy Schools Program	Provides access to the many programs and resources available to help prevent and resolve environmental issues in schools.	http://www.epa.gov/schools/
EPA Toxics Release Inventory	Contains information on toxic chemical releases and other waste management activities reported annually by certain covered industry groups as well as federal facilities.	http://www.epa.gov/tri/
EPA–America's Children & the Environment	Quantitative information from a variety of sources showing trends in levels of environmental contaminants in air, water, food, and soil; concentrations of contaminants measured in the bodies of mothers and children; and childhood diseases that may be influenced by environmental factors	http://www.epa.gov/envirohealth/children/
National Library of Medicine Environmental Health & Toxicology	Includes: TOXNET Hazardous Substances Data Bank (HSDB): broad scope in human and animal toxicity, safety and handling, environmental fate, and more. Scientifically peer-reviewed.	http://sis.nlm.nih.gov/enviro.html

American Academy of Pediatrics, Committee on Environmental Health

Integrated Risk Information System (IRIS): data from the EPA in support of human health risk assessment, focusing on hazard identification and dose-response assessment

Chemical Carcinogenesis Research Information System (CCRIS): carcinogenicity, mutagenicity, tumor promotion, and tumor inhibition data provided by the National Cancer Institute

GENE-TOX: peer-reviewed mutagenicity test data from the EPA

TOXLINE: references to literature on biochemical, pharmacologic, physiologic, and toxicologic effects of drugs and other chemicals

Environmental Mutagen Information Center (EMIC): current and older literature on agents tested for genotoxic activity

Developmental and Reproductive Toxicology and Environmental Teratology Information Center (DART/ETIC): current and older literature on developmental and reproductive toxicology

Toxics Release Inventory (TRI)

ToxSeek

Enviro-Health Links

Tox Town

Household Products Database: information on household products in lay language

LactMed: information abut drugs and lactation

Formulates environmental health policy evaluations for the American Academy of Pediatrics.

www.aap.org/visit/cmte16.htm

(continued on next page)

Table 2 *(continued)*

Name	Description	Location and Contact
Children's Environmental Health Network	National multidisciplinary network to promote a healthy environment and protect the fetus and the child from environmental hazards through a focus on three areas: education of health professionals, research, and federal policy	110 Maryland Avenue NE, Suite 511, Washington, DC 20002 Telephone: (202) 543-4033; Fax: (202) 543-8797; e-mail: cehn@cehn.org http://www.cehn.org;
Children's Health Environmental Coalition	Provides information to parents about the preventable childhood health and developmental problems caused by exposure to toxic substances found in homes, schools and communities.	12300 Wilshire Boulevard, Suite 410, Los Angeles, CA 90025 Telephone: (310) 820-2030; Fax: (310) 820-2070 http://www.checnet.org http://www.checnet.org/healthehouse/virtualhouse/index.asp.
Scorecard	Using authoritative scientific and government data, Scorecard provides information about local environmental information. Ranks and compares the pollution levels in areas across the United States. Also profiles 6800 chemicals, making it easy to find out where they are used and how hazardous they are.	http://scorecard.org
World Health Organization – Protecting the Human Environment	—	http://www.who.int/peh/ For child specific information, see: http://www.who.int/peh/ceh/ For water specific information, see: http://www.who.int/water_sanitation_health/ For chemical specific information, see: http://www.who.int/pcs For information about ionizing radiation, see: http://www.who.int/ionizing_radiation/en/ For information about the air, see: http://www.who.int/peh/air/airindex.htm

For information about ultraviolet radiation, see:
  http://www.who.int/peh-uv/
For information about electro-magnetic fields,
  see: http://www.who.int/peh-emf/en/
For information about occupational health, see:
  http://www.who.int/oeh/index.html
For information about climate, see:
  http://www.who.int/peh/climate/
  climate_and_health.htm
For information about noise, see:
  http://www.who.int/peh/noise/noiseindex.html
For information about solid waste, see:
  http://www.who.int/water_sanitation_health/
  Environmental_sanit/health_care_waste.htm
For information about food safety, see
  http://www.who.int/fsf/
For information about environmental burden of
  disease, see: http://www.who.int/peh/burden/
  burdenindex.htm

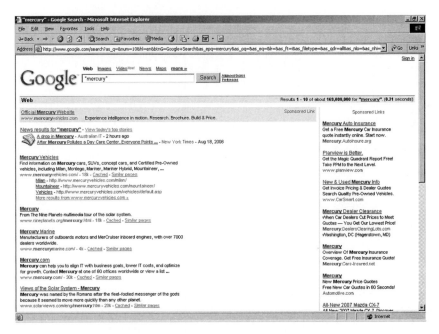

Fig. 2. Screen shot of "mercury" search on Google.com. (Google.com screenshot © Google Inc., reprinted with permission.)

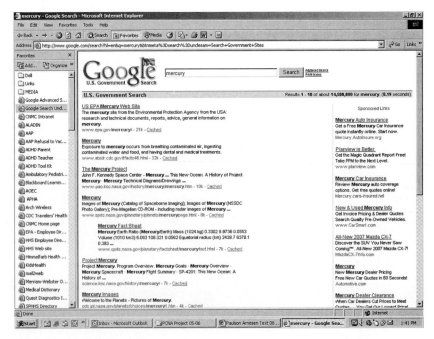

Fig. 3. Screen shot of mercury search on Google.com/ig/usgov. (Google.com screenshot © Google Inc., reprinted with permission.)

There also are important and relevant web pages that one will miss using Google US Government. Any website belonging to an NGO or an international organization such as the World Health Organization will not be retrieved. For example, on the third page of results of a search of the key word "mercury" in the regular Google, one finds the Mercury Policy Project website (www.mercurypolicy.org). The Mercury Policy Project is an NGO that works to promote policies to eliminate mercury uses, reduce the export and trafficking of mercury, and significantly reduce mercury exposures at the local, national, and international levels.

Summary

The World Wide Web contains numerous resources on the effect of the environment on the health of children. The challenge is to identify reliable and up-to-date resources to assist with and enhance research and patient care. The websites listed in this article can serve as initial points of contact to begin researching a new topic (Table 2). From the websites focused on children's health (such as the Children's Environmental Health Network) and from general environmental health databases (such as TOXNET), information on many environmental health issues affecting children can be found. If more information is needed, Internet search engines can identify quickly additional sources of information. By following a few key guidelines for evaluating these resources, new sources of timely, reliable information can be identified.

References

[1] Eitel DR, Yankowitz J, Ely JW. Use of internet technology by obstetricians and family physicians. JAMA 1998;280:1306–7.
[2] Casebeer L, Bennett N, Kristofco R, et al. Physician Internet medical information seeking and on-line continuing education use patterns. J Contin Educ Health Prof 2002;22:33–42.
[3] Bennett NL, Casebeer LL, Kristofco RE, et al. Physicians' internet information-seeking behaviors. J Contin Educ Health Prof 2004;24:31–8.
[4] D'Alessandro DM, Kreiter CD, Peterson MW. An evaluation of information-seeking behaviors of general pediatricians. Pediatrics 2004;113:64–9.
[5] O'Neill ET, Lavoie BF, Bennett R. Trends in the evolution of the public web: 1988-2002. 2003. D-Lib Magazine. 9. Available at: http://www.dlib.org/dlib/april03/lavoie/04lavoie.html. Accessed March 15, 2006.
[6] Gehanno JF, Paris C, Thirion B, et al. Assessment of bibliographic databases performance in information retrieval for occupational and environmental toxicology. Occup Environ Med 1998;55(8):562–6.
[7] Health Summit Working Group. Criteria for assessing the quality of health information on the internet - policy paper. Available at: http://hitiweb.mitretek.org/docs/policy.html. Accessed March 7, 2006.
[8] From: the Infopeople Project: The Infopeople Project is supported by the U.S. Institute of Museum and Library Services under the provisions of the Library Services and Technology Act, administered in California by the State Librarian. Available at: http://infopeople.org/search/tools.html. Accessed January 17, 2006.

PEDIATRIC CLINICS

OF NORTH AMERICA

Pediatr Clin N Am
54 (2007) 155–175

The Challenge Posed to Children's Health by Mixtures of Toxic Waste: The Tar Creek Superfund Site as a Case-Study

Howard Hu, MD, MPH, ScD[a,b,c,]*, James Shine, PhD[b], Robert O. Wright, MD, MPH[a,b,c]

[a]*Department of Environmental Health Sciences, University of Michigan School of Public Health, Room 1518, Vaughan Building (SPH-I), 109 S. Observatory St., Ann Arbor, MI 48109-2029, USA*
[b]*Department of Environmental Health, Harvard School of Public Health, Landmark Center West, 401 Park Drive, Boston, MA 02215, USA*
[c]*Channing Laboratory, Department of Medicine, Brigham and Women's Hospital, Harvard Medical School, 181 Longwood Avenue, Boston, MA 02115, USA*

In the United States, many of the millions of tons of hazardous wastes that have been produced since World War II have accumulated in sites throughout the nation. At first, people were relatively unaware of how dumping chemical wastes might affect public health and the environment. On thousands of properties where such practices were intensive or continuous, the result was uncontrolled or abandoned hazardous waste sites, such as abandoned warehouses and landfills. Citizen concern about the extent of this problem led Congress to establish the Superfund Program in 1980 to locate, investigate, and clean up the worst sites nationwide. The

The work for this publication was made possible by grant number P42-ES05947 and P01 ES012874 from the National Institute of Environmental Health Sciences (NIEHS), NIH and from a STAR Research Assistance Agreement No. RD-83172501 awarded by the U.S. Environmental Protection Agency. It has not been formally reviewed by either the NIEHS or EPA. The views expressed in this document are solely those of the authors and do not necessarily reflect those of either the NIEHS or the EPA. Neither NIEHS nor the EPA endorses any products or commercial services mentioned in this publication.

* Corresponding author. Department of Environmental Health Sciences, University of Michigan School of Public Health, Rm 1518 Vaughan Building (SPH-I), 109 S. Observatory St., Ann Arbor, MI 48109-2029.

E-mail address: howardhu@umich.edu (H. Hu).

0031-3955/07/$ - see front matter © 2007 Elsevier Inc. All rights reserved.
doi:10.1016/j.pcl.2006.11.009
pediatric.theclinics.com

Environmental Protection Agency (EPA) administers the Superfund Program in cooperation with individual states and tribal governments. More than 15,000 such sites have been identified by the EPA across the United States; approximately 1400 of these sites are on the National Priorities List (NPL) and thus are recognized as posing significant potential risks to health [1]. These sites are of a diverse nature, ranging from open-pit lagoons of liquid toxic wastes to abandoned mines, dumped pesticides, aquifers contaminated by leaking gasoline storage tanks, and others. Of the 11 million Americans who are estimated to live within 1 mile of such sites, 3 to 4 million are children under 18 years of age [2].

What are the risks posed to children by toxic or hazardous waste? One of the most vexing challenges that arise when attempting to address this question is the realization that most such waste exists as a complex mixture of many substances. Wastes are rarely segregated; most often, they are dumped together into pits or ponds or added to piles from which human exposure can eventually occur in the form of multiple contaminants in drinking water, airborne dust, crops, and other media. On the other hand, the most of what is known about chemicals and risk has been derived from single-exposure studies, that is, experimental studies in animals of individual toxic agents or in human-population studies that focused on the relationship between individual exposures and adverse outcomes [3]. Such knowledge may not be sufficient to predict the toxicity of mixtures, because evidence is mounting that interactions may occur between toxicants on many levels, and these interactions may, in some cases, have the potential to magnify toxicity greatly.

This article discusses the issue of toxic mixtures and children's health by focusing on the specific example of mining waste at the Tar Creek Superfund Site (TCSS) in Northeast Oklahoma. Mining sites—active, inactive, or abandoned—constitute a major category of Superfund NPL sites that is growing in volume. The Mineral Policy Center estimated in 1995 that, nationwide, there were 557,000 abandoned mines. Most present minimal risks to human health, but many do present risks, and of the 1400 sites on the NPL, 19 were identified as mining "megasites." Overall, the EPA has estimated the cost of cleanup for such sites at more than $24 billion.

At the TCSS, one of the nation's largest such sites, more than 40,000 residents live in a 50-square-mile area filled with mining waste containing lead, manganese, cadmium, and other potentially toxic metals. The TCSS has been the subject of two major on-going studies undertaken by the authors and colleagues with support from the Superfund Basic Research Program and the Center for Children's Environmental Health and Disease Prevention Research at the Harvard School of Public Health. The TCSS serves as an example to discuss issues related to the multiple pathways through which toxic waste mixtures may gain access to the immediate environment of children (or fetuses), factors that may influence absorption of mixtures once ingested or inhaled, the vulnerability of children's developing organs to mixtures, lessons for clinicians, and research needs.

The Tar Creek Superfund Site: mixtures of metals

Background

The TCSS , also known as the Picher Lead/Zinc Mining District of northeastern Oklahoma, was one of the world's largest lead and zinc mining areas. Mining activity in this area began in 1891 and continued until the 1970s, during which time an estimated 1.7 million tons of lead and 8.8 million tons of zinc were produced. It now is one of the largest Superfund sites in the United States, with an area of nearly 50 square miles and estimated costs of remediation and monitoring ranging from $540 million to $61.3 billion [4]. The site was listed on the EPA's Superfund NPL on September 8, 1983. The site is situated in northern Ottawa County, and Tar Creek is the principal drainage system for much of the area, passing through many of the towns before emptying into the Neosho River, one of the two major rivers in northeastern Oklahoma.

Beneath approximately 2500 acres of this site lie around 300 miles of underground tunnels and more than 1300 mineshafts. Thousands of test borings are scattered throughout, many of which are still open. The Boone Formation was the source of the metal ore and also is an aquifer. When mining operations were active, large volumes of water were pumped from the mine workings. When mining operations ceased, the aquifer and mines began refilling, and the native sulfide materials, which had been oxidized by exposure to air, dissolved, creating acid mine water. By 1979, water levels had increased so that the acid mine water began discharging at the surface from several locations, severely impacting Tar Creek.

Much of the surface of the TCSS is an alien landscape notable for mounds of mine tailings, also known as "chat" piles. Some are small, and some are huge; they contain an estimated 165 million tons of waste covering 2900 acres. Many of these tailings are immediately adjacent to residences and schools. Two thirds of the nearly 300 original chat piles have been partially excavated, with the wastes used as fill and road gravel in the district and surrounding areas [4]. Some of the chat was used as fill in the yards of residences and school playgrounds. The piles themselves are an attraction for local residents. Children in particular are drawn to play and bike on the metals-laden tailings, many of which rise 100 or more feet above the ground.

Metals also exist in approximately 800 acres of former flotation ponds that were used to extract metals [5]. Metals from the acid mine water directly contaminate surface water; metals also are available to leach into the Roubidoux aquifer, the regional water supply, by downward migration of acid mine water from the overlying Boone aquifer through abandoned wells and boreholes connecting the two. Metals also can run off during rainfall, and the ever-present Oklahoma winds can blow airborne particles into populated areas. Further dispersion no doubt occurs as vehicles crush the waste used as road gravel, converting it into airborne road dust.

Nine Native American tribes (Cherokee, Eastern Shawnee, Miami, Modoc, Ottawa, Peoria, Quapaw, Seneca Cayuga, and Wyandotte) are represented in the communities located within the boundaries of the TCSS, making ethnic disparities in exposure and "environmental justice" important dimensions to the environmental health problems confronted in this area. Many of the cultural practices of the people who live in this area are heavily dependent on the land, so toxicants that affect the water and vegetation that lie downstream from the heavily contaminated Tri-State Mining District can be expected to affect disproportionately Native Americans, who choose to follow traditional lifestyles, emphasizing consumption of local food and water.

Exposure information

Environmental sampling has demonstrated clearly high levels of lead, cadmium, and iron in various environmental media in the TCSS. For example, in comparison with a control community outside the TCSS, Picher, a town within the TCSS, was found to have mean levels of metals in yard soil that were eight times higher with respect to lead (851 versus 69 mg/kg, respectively), 10 times higher with respect to cadmium (34 versus 3 mg/kg) and more than 10 times higher with respect to iron. Similar results were found for garden soil [6]. In 1996, an EPA emergency response team found that 65% of soil samples from more than 2000 residences in the TCSS had lead concentrations greater than 500 ppm, the action level [7].

Some environmental sampling also has found high levels of manganese. In analyses of mine water by Christenson [8], the median value for levels of manganese was found to be 1870 µg/L with a maximum value of 15,000 µg/L, several orders of magnitude higher than the maximum tolerable level of 50 µg/L set by the EPA for drinking water. Water taken from a sample of 16 Boone boreholes also was found to have high manganese levels, with a mean value of 3318 µg/L and a maximum value of 9800 µg/L [4]. Manganese levels as high as 1900 ppm have been found in sediments along Tar Creek, downstream from the Superfund site in Miami. Well water taken from the Roubidoux aquifer has been found to have manganese levels with a maximum value of 4400 µg/L, with more than 5% of values exceeding 1910 µg/L [4]. In a separate study conducted by the US Geological Survey, water from 14 wells in Ottawa County had manganese levels ranging from 150 to 9800 µg/L with a median value of 3000 µg/L [9].

An initial set of air samples taken near the chat piles at Picher, Oklahoma, did not disclose high levels of toxic metals [10]. Relatively few samples were taken, however, and the possibility remains that airborne metals are a problem further away from the chat piles (eg, where vehicles crush chat used as road gravel into finer, more respirable particles).

Metal mixtures and children: exposure and dose

How might children be exposed to the mixtures of metals that comprise mining waste? The chemistry of acid mine wastes can be complex, and, as the sulfide minerals oxidize, metals potentially can be released into the surrounding environment. Thus, in addition to being a potential primary route of metals exposure, mine tailings also may be a source of bioavailable metals in areas surrounding mine wastes to which humans eventually may be exposed through particles in the water, food, and air.

To understand the risks associated with metals in mine wastes, it is important first to understand the chemical cycling of metals in mining ores as well as the bioavailability of metals in exposure media such as soil, water, indoor dust, and airborne particulates. A challenge is that the chemistry of toxic metals in mine waste piles can be highly dynamic. In parent mine waste, metals typically are present in the form of sulfide minerals, often those that were the targets of metal extraction, such as galena (PbS) and sphalerite (ZnS). The weathering these minerals through exposure to oxygen, moisture, and temperature fluctuations promotes production of acidity and sulfate and the release of metals [11–13]. Some of the dissolved metals released through weathering can migrate offsite with runoff. Mobilized metals also can reprecipitate in situ as secondary minerals such as anglesite ($PbSO_4$), cerrusite ($PbCO_3$) and smithsonite ($ZnCO_3$) and form secondary-mineral rinds on particle surfaces, or they can coprecipitate with or sorb to the surfaces of iron or manganese hydroxides [11,12].

These changes in the geochemical form of the metals are important, because they have a large influence on their bioavailability to humans. Research on metal bioavailability in mine wastes has led to conflicting conclusions. In vitro assessments of bioavailability using sequential extractions and physiologically based extraction tests and in vivo assessments in rats and rabbits have revealed that lead salts such as lead acetate, $PbSO_4$, and lead oxide generally are more bioavailable than PbS and lead-containing mining ores [14–16]. The relatively low bioavailability of metals in sulfides and mine ore has been cited as an explanation for the observation that children in mine-impacted areas have tended to have lower blood lead levels than would be expected given the total lead concentrations in their surroundings, especially as compared with children in urban and smelter-impacted areas [17,18].

Relatively low bioavailability of metals in mining waste also has been shown in plant uptake of metals. Plants grown in mine tailing–amended soils take up a smaller proportion of metals than plants in control areas [19,20] with an effect that is most severe for the metals copper and lead and least severe for the metals zinc and cadmium.

In predicting human exposure, however, this information underplays the reality that secondary mineral phases (ie, metal-containing minerals that have had been weathered, ingested, or otherwise transformed) can be substantially more bioavailable than primary minerals. A significant portion of the lead in mine wastes has been shown to be mobile in environmentally and biologically relevant solutions such as simulated gastric fluid [21]. Furthermore, although many studies have focused solely on lead, other metals (eg, zinc, cadmium, manganese) that frequently occur in mine wastes can have greater environmental mobility than lead and therefore may pose more substantial health risks.

In humans, several epidemiologic studies of communities exposed to lead-contaminated mining waste have failed to find evidence that such exposure contributes significantly to elevations in blood lead levels among children [17,18,22–25].

On the other hand, a number of epidemiologic studies indicate that exposure to mining waste is a major risk factor for increased exposure to metals such as lead.

Gulson and colleagues [26] used isotopic and microscopic characterization techniques to demonstrate that lead in soil samples from the Broken Hill lead mining community in Australia was a major source of lead in house dust and, in all likelihood, of the blood samples of children. Blood lead levels exceeded 20 μg/dL in 20% of the children and 10 μg/dL in 85%. Other investigators used multivariate regression analyses of blood lead levels to come to similar conclusions at other mining sites [27–29].

With respect to the TCSS, the US Public Health Service's Indian Health Service informed the EPA in 1994 that 34% of the 192 Native American children tested from the Tar Creek area had blood lead levels exceeding 10 μg/dL; 15% had blood lead levels above 20 μg/dL [10]. A blood lead survey subsequently conducted in the towns of Quapaw, Picher, and Cardin in 1996 by the Oklahoma State Health Department found that the blood lead levels exceeded the Centers for Disease Control's maximum recommended level of 10 μg/dL in 13.4% (9 of 67), 38.3% (31 of 81), and 63% (10 of 16) of the children tested, respectively [4]. These findings contrast sharply with the statewide average blood lead concentration in children of 2% reported by the Oklahoma State Health Department.

In 1997, baseline blood lead levels among Native American and white children between 1 and 6 years of age residing in Ottawa County were measured as part of a community-based intervention study. the Tribal Efforts Against Lead Project, conducted by researchers at the University of Oklahoma and eight tribes of northeastern Oklahoma. The study area included the five towns constituting the TCSS as well as Miami, the largest city in Ottawa County, and several other nearby small towns. Of the children tested, 21.4% lived in a former mining town. In a multivariate regression analysis, the investigators found that living in one of the former mining towns was associated with a 5.6 odds ratio (95% confidence interval, 1.8–17.8) of having a blood lead greater than 0 µg/dL even after adjusting for mean levels of lead in soil and floor dust, caregivers' education, and hand-to-mouth behaviors [30]. Indices of lead paint (either exterior or interior) did not have a measurable impact on risk of elevated blood lead levels in this population.

A contributing factor in these exposures is that a significant quantity of chat has been dispersed in the community by its removal and use in dirt roads, as an aggregate in concrete, in building foundations, and for sandblasting and landscaping [31]. In particular, there are concerns about the effects of children playing on the chat piles and mobilization of dust from the piles to adjacent residential areas. The issue of windborne transport may be particularly important with respect to children's exposure. Studies have shown that metal concentrations in the fine particles available for windblown transport are enriched relative to the larger particles, with concentrations of lead and zinc as high as 7000 and 55,000 mg/kg, respectively [32]. The highly elevated concentrations of fraction of this size can be important for dust and soil routes of exposure. Soil and dust ingestion may be particularly important in children, for whom hand-to-mouth activity may be more common. Although there is evidence that metals in parent mine wastes have limited bioavailability, exposure data suggest that the metals at the TCSS must have undergone transformations that make them more available for biologic uptake. To develop proper interventions, it thus is imperative to understand better the underlying geochemical cycling that led to these potentially adverse exposures.

Although the potential exists for residents at the TCSS to be also exposed to cadmium, manganese, and other metals, no biologic sampling for metals other than lead has been conducted and published.

Metal mixtures and children: toxicity

Although previous neurodevelopmental research has focused extensively on lead exposure, exposure to other environmental metals, such as arsenic, cadmium, and manganese, may also have toxic effects that have not been well defined in human populations. Furthermore, concurrent exposure to combinations of metals, which is a better reflection of the real world, may have synergistic neurotoxic effects. This situation is particularly critical for populations living near Superfund megasites, because the majority of megasites have multiple contaminants. Former mining communities such as Bunker Hill, Idaho, Leadville, Colorado, and Tar Creek, Oklahoma, among others, are contaminated primarily with metals, including lead, cadmium, arsenic, and manganese. The TCSS site is the focus of the authors' Children's Environmental Health Center research project, and the role of metal mixtures on child development is a predominant theme.

Early-life programming of neurodevelopment

Why are children most vulnerable to neurotoxins? During fetal life and early childhood, neurons must undertake migration, synaptogenesis, selective cell loss, myelination, and a process of selective synaptic pruning before development is complete [33]. Even minor inhibitory or excitatory signals imposed by environmental toxicants at early stages of central nervous system development therefore can cause alterations to subsequent processes. The nature of central nervous system development limits the capacity of the developing brain to compensate for cell loss or disruptions in neural networking caused by neurotoxic chemicals and can lead to reductions in cell numbers [34] or alterations in synaptic architecture [35]. Neurotransmission during the prenatal/early childhood period is a signaling process that determines synaptic and neuronal pruning [36]. Lead interferes with this process by inhibiting depolarization by blocking $Ca++$ channels and by stimulating neurotransmitter release in the absence of an environmental cue [37–41]. Moreover, lead, cadmium, arsenic, and manganese have all been demonstrated to inhibit depolarization-evoked neurotransmitter release. This effect has been shown to be synergistic when these metals are administered as a mixture [42]. By either inhibiting signal transmission or producing spontaneous depolarization in the absence of environmental stimuli, the effect of toxic metals may be to add noise to the neuronal signaling processes that determine synaptic pruning and synaptogenesis. The effects of metals on synaptogenesis and pruning may explain why children are more sensitive to neurotoxins than adults, in whom synaptic architecture is more static and less plastic.

Neurotoxicity of arsenic

Arsenic traditionally has been categorized as a peripheral neurotoxin, producing a clinical picture of severe polyneuropathy. Recent animal studies, however, suggest that this neurotoxicity includes the central nervous system as well. Rodriquez and colleagues [43] demonstrated learning and behavioral deficits in rats exposed to oral arsenic prenatally in maternal drinking water. Arsenic-exposed offspring showed increased spontaneous locomotor activity and increased errors in delayed alternation tasks (a test of memory) compared with unexposed controls. In addition, Nagaraja and Desiraju [44] demonstrated delayed acquisition and extinction of operant behaviors following arsenate exposure in drinking water. Mechanistically, these deficits may be caused by increased oxidative toxicity and changes in neurotransmission. Rao and Avani [45] and Chaudhuri and colleagues [46] demonstrated increased neurotoxic oxidative stress in mouse brains after oral administration of arsenic trioxide. Other investigators have demonstrated changes in levels of neurotransmitters, such as acetylcholine, dopamine, serotonin, and norepinephrine, in the central nervous system after arsenic exposure [35,47,48]. Chattopadhyay and colleagues [49] found that arsenic exposure altered neural networking and led to an increase in reactive oxygen intermediates. The same research team demonstrated that among rats exposed to arsenic during pregnancy, fetal brain neurons underwent apoptotic changes and neuronal necrosis [47]. Recent epidemiologic literature also confirms that environmental levels of arsenic exposure may produce neurocognitive deficits in children [50]. Calderon and colleagues [51] demonstrated that urinary arsenic levels inversely predicted verbal IQ among 39 children living proximal to a smelter, even after adjusting for blood lead. Recently, Wasserman and colleagues [52] conducted a cohort study of children that demonstrated a strong adverse effect of elevated drinking water arsenic levels on IQ after adjusting for covariates.

Neurotoxicity of manganese

Unlike arsenic and lead, manganese is a toxic metal but also is an essential nutrient [53]. Nutritional deficiencies of manganese, therefore, are possible but extremely rare. Adult workers exposed to high levels of air manganese levels have memory loss, anxiety, behavior changes, and sleep disturbances [54–56]. In its final stages, manganism leads to a Parkinsonian-like syndrome. The primary mechanisms of manganese neurotoxicity are not well understood but seem to involve increased oxidative damage to neuronal cells [57–59]. With respect to potential developmental neurotoxicity, Tran and colleagues [60] demonstrated that increased dietary manganese supplements fed to lactating dams was associated with decreased striatal dopamine levels 1 month following cessation of supplements as well as with significant increases in passive avoidance errors among animals who received manganese [61]. In adults living in Greece, abnormal neurologic scores were associated with higher manganese concentrations in hair and in water [62]. Santos-Burgoa and colleagues [63] reported a significant inverse association between blood manganese levels and Mini-Mental Status Examination scores among adults living proximal to a manganese-mining district in central Mexico. In Chinese children, exposure to elevated manganese concentrations in drinking water was associated with lower scores on tests of short-term memory, manual dexterity, and visual-perceptual speed [64]. The present authors recently reported a child with manganism (blood manganese, 3.8 µg/dL) from a private well-water source who had a normal full-scale IQ but deficits in verbal, visual, and general memory indices [65]. Using the McCarthy General Cognitive Index test at age 5 years, Takser and colleagues [66] reported deficits in memory, attention, and psychomotor indices associated with elevated umbilical cord manganese levels. More recently, Wasserman and colleagues [67] found inverse associations between water manganese levels and IQ among 10-year-old children.

Neurotoxicity of cadmium

Like arsenic and manganese, cadmium has neurotoxic properties, but population-based studies in children are lacking, although some research has been reported. The neurotoxicity of cadmium in children was investigated in several studies in the 1970s and 1980s but has received little attention since. In most of these studies, the biomarker of exposure was the concentration of cadmium in hair. In case-control studies in which the hair concentration of cadmium of a clinically defined group was compared with that of a reference group, higher concentrations were reported in mentally retarded children [68,69] and in children who had learning difficulties or dyslexia [70,71] but not in children who had autism [72,73] or any of several neuropsychiatric diagnoses (motor, perceptual, speech, or attention disorders) [74]. In cohort studies, Thatcher and colleagues [75,76] reported that the concentration of cadmium in hair was significantly inversely related to adjusted IQ scores, particularly verbal IQ, and to visual evoked potentials [77]. Marlowe and colleagues [78,79] reported associations between increased hair cadmium and children's performance on visual-motor tasks. Marlowe and colleagues [80] also reported that lead and cadmium acted synergistically in impair children's classroom behavior.

The neurotoxicity of lead

The literature supporting the neurodevelopmental toxicity of lead is extensive, and a comprehensive summary is beyond the scope of this article. Although controversy still exists regarding the levels at which lead toxicity manifests clinically, there is widespread acceptance that lead is neurotoxic. Lead exposure can occur pre- and postnatally, because lead freely crosses the placenta [81]. Levels of lead circulating in maternal blood provide information about in utero exposure to the fetus [82]. Several investigators have reported inverse associations between infants' scores on tests of cognitive and motor development and an index of fetal lead exposure such as umbilical cord blood concentration [83,84] or maternal blood lead during pregnancy [85]. Neonatal (10-day) blood lead levels, interpreted as an index of prenatal exposures, were associated with worse performance at age 4 years on all scales of the Kaufman-Assessment Battery for Children [86]. Bellinger and colleagues [87] demonstrated that the deficits of children who had higher prenatal exposures (cord-blood lead levels of 10 to 25 µg/dL) persisted until 2 years of age, despite postnatal exposures that were comparable with those of children who had lower prenatal exposures. The toxicity of lead in combination with other metals is largely unexplored, particularly in humans.

Metal mixtures and neurodevelopment

Data on chemical mixtures in humans are limited to only a few studies [88–90]. Animal studies have demonstrated increased spontaneous motor activity among rats with joint manganese/lead exposures relative to those with only one metal [91,92]. In studies of conditioned avoidance responses, lead plus manganese decreased learning more than either lead or manganese alone [91]. Gestational exposure to lead and manganese combined reduces birth weight and brain weight more than either metal alone [92].

Coadministration of lead and manganese has been demonstrated to increase brain lead levels approximately threefold [91,93]. As with joint manganese and lead exposure, rats jointly exposed to arsenic and lead have higher levels of lead in the midbrain and hippocampus than animals exposed to lead alone [94]. In addition, multiplicatively greater changes in monoaminergic neurotransmitter levels occur in the brains of rats exposed to lead and arsenic jointly than in rates exposed to either metal alone [94]. Rodriguez and colleagues [43] administered mining waste containing lead, manganese, and arsenic to rats in their diets and found elevations of both arsenic and manganese in rat brains relative to controls with single-metal exposures. The three-metal concentrations were highly correlated and predicted decreases in dopaminergic neurotransmitter release following depolarization.

Recently, the present authors conducted a study of arsenic/manganese exposure and IQ among sixth grade children living in the TCSS [95]. Hair metal levels were used as an index of exposure. An inverse association existed for verbal and full-scale IQ with hair arsenic and hair manganese. In linear regression models both hair arsenic and hair manganese were significantly associated with both full-scale and verbal IQ. Hair lead and hair cadmium did not significantly predict any IQ test score. The effect of both hair arsenic and hair manganese remained after adjusting for maternal education and for gender. Hair arsenic and manganese were highly correlated ($r^2 = 0.42$) and could not be entered into a single model because of colinearity. There was evidence of an interaction, however. When the data were dichotomized by the median values of hair arsenic and hair manganese, only subjects who jointly had elevated hair arsenic and manganese had lowered IQ test scores, suggesting that joint exposures may be most toxic.

Metal mixtures: potential interventions

Nutrition and toxic metals

There is substantial variability in biomarkers of internal dose among children exposed to metals. Multiple factors contribute to this variance. Behavioral factors such as hand-to- mouth activity, differences in environmental levels even among children living in the same neighborhood, size differences in children of the same age, and variability in genetic susceptibility all likely play a role. Many of these factors cannot be modified or are difficult to measure, limiting their clinical utility for pediatricians caring for high-risk children. One of the few factors that can be modified clinically is diet. A substantial body of evidence has demonstrated that body stores of essential nutrients, such as calcium, zinc, and iron are generally inversely related to the absorption of toxic divalent metals such as lead, manganese, and cadmium.

Calcium and toxic metal absorption

Calcium influences the remobilization of lead from bone and also the absorption of lead in the gut. Animals fed a calcium-deficient diet have higher blood lead levels than control animals with identical lead exposures through water [96,97]. The inverse association between dietary calcium intake and blood lead concentrations also has been demonstrated in large cohort studies, such as the National Health and Nutrition Examination Study [98] and even in early experimental studies [99,100]. This large body of evidence eventually led to a randomized, controlled trial of calcium supplementation in the formula of infants to prevent lead poisoning [101]. Although the study did not demonstrate a significant effect in preventing lead poisoning, the sample size was relatively small (103 infants total), and calcium supplementation was discontinued at 1 year of age and not continued to the peak age of lead poisoning (1.5–3 years of age). The authors' research group has demonstrated that calcium supplementation will decrease lead exposure during lactation [102]. Calcium absorption also is inversely associated with other divalent metals such as cadmium and manganese that may be transferred in breast milk and are found in bone [103–105]. Low dietary calcium intake has been associated with increased manganese absorption. Yasui and colleagues [106] found a significant increase in bone concentrations of manganese when rats were fed a low-calcium diet. Similarly, Murphy and colleagues [107] found a fourfold increase in serum manganese concentrations in rats fed a low-calcium, normal-manganese diet. Cadmium absorption also is inversely associated with dietary calcium [108,109]. In addition, low dietary calcium alters the tissue distribution of cadmium, increasing brain levels [110]. A low-calcium diet coupled with cadmium exposure increased bone demineralization during pregnancy and lactation [111]. Sari and colleagues [112], studied the effect of calcium supplementation in suckling rats through gavage supplementation of breast milk with cow's milk and found reductions in body cadmium. Walter and colleagues [113] found a similar effect of calcium supplements reducing cadmium retention in rats.

Iron and toxic metals absorption

In addition to inverse associations between dietary calcium intake and absorption of lead, manganese, and cadmium, there is substantial evidence that iron deficiency increases the absorption of these three metals. During iron deficiency, regulatory mechanisms cause an increase in the percentage of ingested iron that is absorbed [96]. Barton and colleagues [114] suggested that the effects of iron deficiency on lead absorption are mediated through a common absorptive pathway for both metals. In clinical studies, an inverse association between dietary iron and blood lead was found in urban Baltimore children by Hammad [115]. Similarly, the present authors' research group recently found an association between iron deficiency and low-level lead poisoning in children [116,117]. Other clinical studies also have demonstrated that high body iron stores are associated with decreased blood lead levels [82,118]. Iron deficiency also increases manganese absorption [119]. Intracellular uptake of manganese occurs with cotransport of iron [58]. Animal studies clearly demonstrate that iron deficiency increases manganese absorption independent of body manganese stores [119,120]. Similarly, an inverse association between serum ferritin levels and manganese absorption has been demonstrated in humans [121]. Body iron status also seems to modify cadmium absorption. Groten and colleagues [122] showed that low dietary iron content was associated with increased intestinal uptake of cadmium in rats. Increases in dietary cadmium absorption have been inversely associated with serum ferritin levels in both mice and humans [123–125].

Selenium and arsenic

Arsenic metabolism and toxicity are more closely related to a different essential mineral, selenium. Selenium is an essential trace element involved in antioxidant defense, thyroid function, and immune function. Although clinically apparent selenium-deficiency diseases have been reported, evidence is emerging that preclinical deficiency also can cause adverse health effects. Available data indicate that selenium antagonizes arsenic-induced disease. The proposed mechanisms of this interaction include the increased biliary excretion and direct interaction/precipitation of selenium and arsenic and their effects on zinc finger protein function, cellular signaling, and methylation pathways [126]. Maintaining body stores of selenium may be critical in preventing the neurotoxicity of arsenic.

Other interventions

The previous section highlights the potential benefits of nutrient supplementation in preventing the absorption of toxic metals. Other interventions include chelation for lead-poisoned children and reducing environmental hazard. Chelation for low-level lead poisoning (blood lead levels < 40 μg/dL) has not been demonstrated to be effective in preventing poorer cognitive outcomes [127]. Prevention measures therefore have become the focus of most clinical efforts, but such measures have been largely unsuccessful when tested in randomized, controlled trials [101]. Attempts to reduce dust loading in the housing of high-risk children have been similarly disappointing. A systematic review of randomized, controlled trials of low-cost, dust-control interventions to determine the effect of lead hazard control on children's blood lead concentration found no significant differences in mean change in blood lead concentration by group assignment [128]. A randomized trial of soil abatement in urban children conducted in the late 1980s and early 1990s also did not find a significant effect on children's blood lead levels. With respect to soil abatement at Superfund sites in which lead paint may be a less dominant source, there are no randomized trials similar to that of Weitzman and colleagues [129]. Lanphear and colleagues [130], however, did find a significant decrease in blood lead levels associated with soil abatement in an observational study conducted in a population adjacent to a lead/arsenic smelter. Given the ethical ramifications of a nontreatment arm and the inability to blind soil-abatement measures, a true randomized, controlled trial of soil abatement within a Superfund mining megasite is unlikely to be conducted. The weight of the existing evidence therefore suggests that soil abatement is beneficial at such sites.

Given that few studies have demonstrated effective measures that reduce blood lead levels, removing lead from a child's environment is probably the most effective public health measure. Clinicians, however, are most often faced with individual children who are either lead poisoned or who live in a known high-risk environment. Measures to reduce dust exposure, such as focused cleaning around windowsills and doormats to minimize dust lead loading, should be encouraged. Although more costly, ideally a household should use a vacuum equipped with a high-efficiency particulate air filter; otherwise there is risk of spreading the dust beyond the area of cleaning. Cleaning should involve vacuuming of major horizontal surfaces (floors, windowsills, and furniture) as well as mopping. Hand washing, particularly after outdoor play, should be emphasized. Dust and soil are likely sources of lead and also of multiple metals in children living near former mining communities, Furthermore, nutritional interventions aimed at preventing lead absorption probably will prevent the absorption/toxicity of other toxic metals, such as manganese, cadmium, and possibly arsenic. Nutritional interventions have the added benefit of reducing the overall prevalence of iron deficiency anemia or calcium deficiency, which may have their own neurotoxic effects. Nutritional supplements of iron, zinc, and calcium therefore may work both directly and indirectly to improve neurodevelopmental outcomes in at-risk children and should be encouraged by clinicians.

Metal mixtures: summary and lessons for clinicians

Much is known about the toxicity of individual environmental risk factors, but little is known about their potential interactions in mixtures, which, unfortunately, represent the vast majority of exposures stemming from real-world hazards such as toxic waste sites. This article has used the case study of the TCSS, the focus of the authors' research and an area where thousands of residents, including children, live amid mounds of chat mining waste, to discuss and illustrate the challenges in assessing and controlling risks from mixtures of toxic metals. The first issues that must be evaluated are the various routes of exposure and bioavailability (the ability of metals to be absorbed) once mining waste dusts are ingested or inhaled. The evidence that such exposures are occurring at the TCSS with resulting doses of lead and other metals is high, although the extent remains to be clarified. The neurotoxicity of lead at low levels is now well established, and the neurotoxicity to children of low-level exposures to arsenic, manganese, and other metals is of great concern and the subject of ongoing research. Animal studies and preliminary human studies suggest that synergy (metal–metal interactions that multiply risk) may occur also.

While this research progresses, there are some low-risk interventions with high potential benefits that make particular sense for communities exposed to mixtures of metals (such as mining waste): focused cleaning of surfaces with a high-efficiency particulate air vacuum cleaner, frequent hand washing, and nutritional supplementation using foods and/or supplements containing iron, zinc, calcium, and possibly selenium.

When confronted by patients or communities that are potentially affected by hazards such as metal mixtures in mining waste, clinicians need to be able to access and interpret a diverse array of informational sources on exposures, potential toxicity, methods of environmental and medical monitoring, and best practices. A growing amount of such information is becoming available on Web sites maintained by the government, nongovernmental organizations, and academic institutions. Table 1 provides a list of suggested Internet resources related to toxic wastes and health. The availability of the

Table 1
Examples of internet-based resources related to toxic metals, wastes and health

Description	Website
Agency for Toxic Substances and Disease Registry (ATSDR): a government agency that studies health effects of toxic waste	http://www.atsdr.cdc.gov
ATSDR Case Studies in Environmental Medicine: information for clinicians on specific exposures	http://www.atsdr.cdc.gov/HEC/CSEM/ csem.html
ATSDR Chemical Mixtures Program	http://www.atsdr.cdc.gov/mixtures.html
Center for Children's Environmental Health and Disease Prevention Research at the Harvard School of Public Health: metal mixtures and children's health	http://www.hsph.harvard.edu/niehs/children
Dartmouth Toxic Metals Research Program	http://www.dartmouth.edu/~toxmetal/ HM.shtml
EPA Superfund Program (general description)	http://www.epa.gov/superfund
EPA Search Engine:(for finding toxic waste sites in a community	http://cfpub.epa.gov/supercpad/cursites/ srchsites.cfm
Metals Epidemiology Research Group: a Harvard–University of Michigan research collaboration on metals toxicity	http://www.hsph.harvard.edu/merg
National Center for Environmental Health (NCEH): a government agency that addresses broad environmental health issues	http://www.cdc.gov/nceh

Internet and the growing sophistication of search engines make such information more easily available than ever before, but integrating and synthesizing the information to arrive at specific clinical recommendations can be challenging, even for clinicians trained in environmental health and environmental medicine, and particularly in a setting in which mixtures prevail and in which many unknowns exist.

References

[1] Landrigan PJ, Suk WA, Amler RW. Chemical wastes, children's health, and the Superfund Basic Research Program. Environ Health Perspect 1999;107:423–7.

[2] Browner C. Environmental health threats to children. EPA 175-F-96–001. Washington, DC: U.S. Environmental Protection Agency; 1996.

[3] Carpenter DO, Arcaro KF, Bush B, et al. Human health and chemical mixtures: an overview. Environ Health Perpec 1998;106(Suppl 6):1263–70.

[4] Oklahoma Office of the Secretary of Environment. Governor Frank Keating's Tar Creek Superfund Task Force Final Report; 2000.

[5] U.S. EPA, Region 6. Superfund fact sheet: Tar Creek Site, soils remediation update, October 7, 2002. Tar Creek (Ottawa County) Oklahoma. Dallas (TX): U.S. Environmental Protection Agency; 2002.

[6] Ecology and Environment, Inc. Baseline human health risk assessment of residential exposures. August 1996.

[7] U.S. EPA, Region 6. Record of decision: residential areas, operable unit 2, Tar Creek Superfund Site, Ottawa County, Oklahoma. Dallas (TX): U.S. Environmental Protection Agency; August 1997. Available at: http://www.epa.gov/region6/6st/pdffiles/rod-tarcreekou2.pdf. Accessed April 19, 2003.

[8] Christenson S. Contamination of wells completed in the Roubidoux aquifer by abandoned zinc and lead mines, Ottawa County, Oklahoma. Oklahoma City: U.S. Geological Survey, Water-Resources Investigations Report 1995; 95-4150.

[9] US Geological Survey. Project title: assessment of ground-water flow and recharge in the Boone aquifer in Ottawa County, Oklahoma, 2002. Available at: http://ok.water.usgs.gov/proj/boone.aquifer.html. Accessed April 25, 2003.

[10] US EPA Region 6. Five year review. Tar Creek Superfund Site, Ottawa County, Oklahoma. Dallas (TX): U.S. Environmental Protection Agency; April 1994.

[11] Al TA, Blowes DW, Martin CJ, et al. Aqueous geochemistry and analysis of pyrite surfaces in sulfide-rich mine tailings. Geochim Cosmochim Acta 1997;61(12):2353–66.

[12] Martin CJ, Al TA, Cabri LJ. Surface analysis of particles in mine tailings by time-of-flight laser-ionization mass spectrometry (TOF-LIMS). Environmental Geology 1997;32(2):107–13.

[13] Stanton MR. The role of weathering in trace metal distributions in subsurface samples from the Mayday Mine Dump near Silverton, Colorado. Proceedings from the Fifth International Conference on Acid Rock Drainage, Denver (CO): Society for Mining, Metallurgy, and Exploration Inc., 2000.

[14] Rieuwerts JS, Farago ME, Cikrt M, et al. Differences in lead bioavailability between a smelting and a mining area. Water Air Soil Pollut 2000;122:203–29.

[15] Oomen AG, Tolls J, Sips AJAM, et al. Lead speciation in artificial human digestive fluid. Arch Environ Contam Toxicol 2003;44(1):107–15.

[16] Ruby MV. Bioavailability of soil-borne chemicals: abiotic assessment tools. Human and Ecological Risk Assessment 2004;10(4):647–56.

[17] Steele MI, Beck BD, Murphy BL, et al. Assessing the contribution from lead in mining wastes to blood lead. Regulatory Toxicology and Pharmacology 1990;11:158–90.

[18] Bierre B, Berglund M, Harsbo K, et al. Blood lead concentrations of Swedish preschool children in a community with high lead levels from mine waste in soil and dust. Scand J Work Environ Health 1993;19:154–61.

[19] Jung MC, Thornton I. Environmental contamination and seasonal variation of metals in soils, plants and waters in the paddy fields around a Pb-Zn mine in Korea. Sci Total Environ 1997;198(2):105–21.

[20] Bunzl K, Trautmannsheimer M, Schramel P, et al. Availability of arsenic, copper, lead, thallium, and zinc to various vegetables grown in slag-contaminated soils. J Environ Qual 2001;30(3):934–9.

[21] Gasser UG, Walker WJ, Dahlgren RA, et al. Lead release from smelter and mine waste impacted materials under simulated gastric conditions and relation to speciation. Environ Sci Technol 1996;30(3):761–9.

[22] Danse IH, Garb LG, Moore RH. Blood lead surveys of communities in proximity to lead-containing mill tailings. Am Ind Hyg Assoc J 1995;56(4):384–93.

[23] Bornschein RL, Clark CS, Grote J, et al. Soil lead-blood lead relationships in a former lead mining town. Environ Geochem Health 1989;9:149–60.

[24] Colorado Department of Health. Leadville Metals Exposure Study: final report. Division of Disease Control and Environmental Epidemiology, Denver (CO): Colorado Department of Health jointly with the U.S. Agency for Toxic Substances and Disease Registry; 1990.

[25] Woodward-Clyde Consultants. Trends in children's blood lead levels and sources of environmental lead exposures. Report for ASARCO. Leadville (CO): Project No. 22909K; 1993.

[26] Gulson BL, Davis JJ, Mizon KJ, et al. Lead bioavailability in the environment of children: blood lead levels in children can be elevated in a mining community. Arch Environ Health 1994;49:326–31.

[27] Cook M, Chappell WR, Hoffman RE, et al. Assessment of blood lead levels in children living in historical mining and smelting community. Am J Epidemiol 1993;137:447–55.

[28] Dutkiewicz T, Sokolowska D, Kulka E. Health risk assessment in children exposed to lead compounds in the vicinity of mine-smelter plant "Orzel Bialy". Pol J Occup Med Environ Health 1993;6:71–8.

[29] Murgueytio AM, Gregory Evans R, Roberts D. Relationship between soil and dust lead in a lead mining area and blood lead levels. J Expo Anal Environ Epidemiol 1998;8:173–86.

[30] Malcoe LH, Lynch RA, Kegler MC, et al. Lead sources, behaviors, and socioeconomic factors in relation to blood lead of Native American and white children: a community-based assessment of a former mining area. Environ Health Perspect 2002;110(Suppl 2): 221–31.

[31] Perry PM, Pavlik JW, Sheets RW, et al. Lead, cadmium, and zinc concentrations in plaster and mortar from structures in Jasper and Newton Counties, Missouri (Tri-State Mining District). Sci Total Environ 2005;336(1–3):275–81.

[32] Datin DL, and Cates DA. Sampling and metal analysis of chat piles in the Tar Creek Superfund Site. Oklahoma City (OK): Oklahoma Department of Environmental Quality; 2002. Available at: http://www.deq.state.ok.us//lpdnew/Tarcreek/TarCreekChatPaper.pdf. Accessed April 9, 2006.

[33] Faustman EM, Silbernagel SM, Fenske RA, et al. Mechanisms underlying children's susceptibility to environmental toxicants. Environ Health Perspect 2000;108(Suppl 1):13–21.

[34] Bayer SA. Cellular aspects of brain development. Neurotoxicology 1989;10:307–20.

[35] Bressler J, Kim KA, Chakraborti T, et al. Molecular mechanisms of lead neurotoxicity. Neurochem Res 1999;24:595–600.

[36] Bressler JP, Goldstein GW. Mechanisms of lead neurotoxicity. Biochem Pharmacol 1991; 41:479–84.

[37] Suszkiw J, Toth G, Murawsky M, et al. Effects of Pb2+ and Cd2+ on acetylcholine release and Ca2+ movements in synaptosomes and subcellular fractions from rat brain and Torpedo electric organ. Brain Res 1984;323:31–46.

[38] Minnema DJ, Greenland RD, Michaelson IA. Effect of in vitro inorganic lead on dopamine release from superfused rat striatal synaptosomes. Toxicol Appl Pharmacol 1986;84: 400–11.

[39] Minnema DJ, Michaelson IA. Differential effects of inorganic lead and delta-aminolevulinic acid in vitro on synaptosomal gamma-aminobutyric acid release. Toxicol Appl Pharmacol 1986;86:437–47.

[40] Minnema DJ, Michaelson IA, Cooper GP. Calcium efflux and neurotransmitter release from rat hippocampal synaptosomes exposed to lead. Toxicol Appl Pharmacol 1988;92: 351–7.

[41] Lasley SM, Gilbert ME. Presynaptic glutamatergic function in dentate gyrus in vivo is diminished by chronic exposure to inorganic lead. Brain Res 1996;736:125–34.

[42] Rodriguez VM, Dufour L, Carrizales L, et al. Effects of oral exposure to mining waste on in vivo dopamine release from rat striatum. Environ Health Perspect 1998;106:487–91.

[43] Rodriguez VM, Carrizales L, Mendoza MS, et al. Effects of sodium arsenite exposure on development and behavior in the rat. Neurotoxicol Teratol 2002;24:743–50.

[44] Nagaraja TN, Desiraju T. Effects on operant learning and brain acetylcholine esterase activity in rats following chronic inorganic arsenic intake. Hum Exp Toxicol 1994;13:353–6.

[45] Rao M, Avani G. Arsenic induced free radical toxicity in brain of mice. Indian J Exp Biol 2004;42:495–8.

[46] Chaudhuri AN, Basu S, Chattopadhyay S, et al. Effect of high arsenic content in drinking water on rat brain. Indian J Biochem Biophys 1999;36:51–4.

[47] Chattopadhyay S, Bhaumik S, Purkayastha M, et al. Apoptosis and necrosis in developing brain cells due to arsenic toxicity and protection with antioxidants. Toxicol Lett 2002;136: 65–76.

[48] Nagaraja TN, Desiraju T. Regional alterations in the levels of brain biogenic amines, glutamate, GABA, and GAD activity due to chronic consumption of inorganic arsenic in developing and adult rats. Bull Environ Contam Toxicol 1993;50:100–7.

[49] Chattopadhyay S, Bhaumik S, Nag Chaudhury A, et al. Arsenic induced changes in growth development and apoptosis in neonatal and adult brain cells in vivo and in tissue culture. Toxicol Lett 2002;128:73–84.

[50] Tsai SY, Chou HY, The HW, et al. The effects of chronic arsenic exposure from drinking water on the neurobehavioral development in adolescence. Neurotoxicology 2003;24: 747–53.

[51] Calderon J, Navarro ME, Jimenez-Capdeville ME, et al. Exposure to arsenic and lead and neuropsychological development in Mexican children. Environ Res 2001;85:69–76.

[52] Wasserman GA, Liu X, Parvez F, et al. Water arsenic exposure and children's intellectual function in Araihazar, Bangladesh. Environ Health Perspect 2004;112:1329–33.

[53] McMillan DE. A brief history of the neurobehavioral toxicity of manganese: some unanswered questions. Neurotoxicology 1999;20:499–507.

[54] Rodier J. Manganese poisoning in Moroccan miners. Br J Ind Med 1955;12:21–35.

[55] Sassine MP, Mergler D, Bowler R, et al. Manganese accentuates adverse mental health effects associated with alcohol use disorders. Biol Psychiatry 2002;51:909–21.

[56] Wennberg A, Iregren A, Struwe G, et al. Manganese exposure in steel smelters a health hazard to the nervous system. Scand J Work Environ Health 1991;17:255–62.

[57] Aschner M, Aschner JL. Manganese neurotoxicity: cellular effects and blood-brain barrier transport. Neurosci Biobehav Rev 1991;15:333–40.

[58] Verity MA. Manganese neurotoxicity: a mechanistic hypothesis. Neurotoxicology 1999;20: 489–97.

[59] Zheng W, Ren S, Graziano JH. Manganese inhibits mitochondrial aconitase: a mechanism of manganese neurotoxicity. Brain Res 1998;799:334–42.

[60] Tran TT, Chowanadisai W, Crinella FM, et al. Effect of high dietary manganese intake of neonatal rats on tissue mineral accumulation, striatal dopamine levels, and neurodevelopmental status. Neurotoxicology 2002;23:635–43.

[61] Tran TT, Chowanadisai W, Lonnerdal B, et al. Effects of neonatal dietary manganese exposure on brain dopamine levels and neurocognitive functions. Neurotoxicology 2002;23: 645–51.

[62] Kondakis XG, Makris N, Leotsinidis M, et al. Possible health effects of high manganese concentration in drinking water. Arch Environ Health 1989;44:175–8.

[63] Santos-Burgoa C, Rios C, Mercado LA, et al. Exposure to manganese: health effects on the general population, a pilot study in central Mexico. Environ Res 2001;85:90–104.

[64] He P, Liu DH, Zhang GQ. [Effects of high-level-manganese sewage irrigation on children's neurobehavior]. Zhonghua Yu Fang Yi Xue Za Zhi 1994;28:216–8.

[65] Woolf A, Wright R, Amarasiriwardena C, et al. A child with chronic manganese exposure from drinking water. Environ Health Perspect 2002;110:613–6.

[66] Takser L, Mergler D, Hellier G, et al. Manganese, monoamine metabolite levels at birth, and child psychomotor development. Neurotoxicology 2003;24:667–74.

[67] Wasserman GA, Liu X, Parvez F, et al. Water manganese exposure and children's intellectual function in Araihazar, Bangladesh. Environ Health Perspect 2006;114(1):124–9.

[68] Marlowe M, Errera J, Jacobs J. Increased lead and cadmium burdens among mentally retarded children and children with borderline intelligence. Am J Ment Defic 1983;87:477–83.

[69] Jiang HM, Guo H, Zhu H. Clinical significance of hair cadmium content in the diagnosis of mental retardation of children. Chin Med J 1990;103:331–4.

[70] Pihl RO, Parkes M. Hair element content in learning disabled children. Science 1977;198: 204–6.

[71] Capel ID, Pinnock MH, Dorrell HM, et al. Comparison of concentrations of some trace, bulk, and toxic metals in the hair of normal and dyslexic children. Clin Chem 1981;27: 879–91.

[72] Shearer TR, Larson K, Neuschwander J, et al. Minerals in the hair and nutrient intake of autistic children. J Autism Dev Disord 1982;12(1):25–34.

[73] Wecker L, Miller SB, Cochran SR, et al. Trace element concentrations in hair from autistic children. J Ment Defic Res 1985;29:15–22.

[74] Gillberg C, Noren JG, Wahlstrom J, et al. Heavy metals and neuropsychiatric disorders in six-year-old children. Acta Paedopsychiatr 1982;48:253–63.

[75] Thatcher RW, Lester ML, McAlaster R, et al. Effects of low levels of cadmium and lead on cognitive functioning in children. Arch Environ Health 1982;37:159–66.

[76] Thatcher RW, McAlaster R, Lester ML. Evoked potentials related to hair cadmium and lead in children. Ann N Y Acad Sci 1984;425:384–90.

[77] Bonithon-Kopp C, Huel G, Moreau T, et al. Prenatal exposure to lead and cadmium and psychomotor development of the child at 6 years. Neurobehav Toxicol Teratol 1986;8(3): 307–10.

[78] Stellern J, Marlowe M, Cossairt A, et al. Low lead and cadmium levels and childhood visual-perception development. Percept Mot Skills 1983;56(2):539–44.

[79] Marlowe M, Stellern J, Errera J, et al. Main and interaction effects of metal pollutants on visual-motor performance. Arch Environ Health 1985;40:221–5.

[80] Marlowe M, Cossairt A, Moon C, et al. Main and interaction effects of metallic toxins on classroom behavior. J Abnorm Child Psychol 1985;13:185–98.

[81] Goyer RA. Results of lead research: prenatal exposure and neurological consequences. Environ Health Perspect 1996;104:1050–4.

[82] Graziano JH, Popovac D, Factor-Litvak P, et al. Determinants of elevated blood lead during pregnancy in a population surrounding a lead smelter in Kosovo, Yugoslavia. Environ Health Perspect 1990;89:95–100.

[83] Bellinger D, Leviton A, Waternaux C, et al. Longitudinal analyses of pre-and postnatal lead exposure and early cognitive development. N Engl J Med 1987;316:1037–43.

[84] Wasserman GA, Graziano JH, Factor-Litvak P, et al. Consequences of lead exposure and iron supplementation on childhood development at age 4 years. Neurotoxicol Teratol 1994; 16:233–40.

[85] Dietrich KN, Krafft KM, Bornschein RL, et al. Low-level fetal lead exposure effect on neurobehavioral development in early infancy. Pediatrics 1987;80:721–30.

[86] Dietrich KN, Succop PA, Berger OG, et al. Lead exposure and the cognitive development of urban preschool children: the Cincinnati Lead Study cohort at age 4 years. Neurotoxicol Teratol 1991;13:203–11.

[87] Bellinger D, Sloman J, Leviton A, et al. Low-level lead exposure and children's cognitive function in the preschool years. Pediatrics 1991;87:219–27.

[88] Delves HT, Clayton BE, Bicknell J. Concentration of trace metals in the blood of children. Br J Prev Soc Med 1973;27:100–7.

[89] Joselow MM, Tobias E, Koehler R, et al. Manganese pollution in the city environment and its relationship to traffic density. Am J Public Health 1978;68:557–60.

[90] Zielhuis RL, del Castilho P, Herber RF, et al. Levels of lead and other metals in human blood: suggestive relationships, determining factors. Environ Health Perspect 1978;25:103–9.

[91] Chandra AV, Ali MM, Saxena DK, et al. Behavioral and neurochemical changes in rats simultaneously exposed to manganese and lead. Arch Toxicol 1981;49:49–56.

[92] Chandra SV, Murthy RC, Saxena DK, et al. Effects of pre- and postnatal combined exposure to Pb and Mn on brain development in rats. Ind Health 1983;21:273–9.

[93] Malhotra KM, Murthy RC, Srivastava RS, et al. Concurrent exposure of lead and manganese to iron-deficient rats: effect on lipid peroxidation and contents of some metals in the brain. J Appl Toxicol 1984;4:22–5.

[94] Mejia JJ, Diaz-Barriga F, Calderon J, et al. Effects of lead-arsenic combined exposure on central monoaminergic systems. Neurotoxicol Teratol 1997;19:489–97.

[95] Wright RO, Amarasiriwardena C, Woolf AD, et al. Neuropsychological correlates of hair arsenic, manganese, and cadmium levels in school-age children residing near a hazardous waste site. Neurotoxicology 2006;27(2):210–6.

[96] Mahaffey-Six K, Goyer R. The influence of iron deficiency on tissue content and toxicity of ingested lead in the rat. J Lab Clin Med 1972;79:128–36.

[97] Barltrop D, Khoo HE. The influence of dietary minerals and fat on the absorption of lead. Sci Total Environ 1976;6:265–73.

[98] Mahaffey KR, Gartside PS, Glueck CJ. Blood lead levels and dietary calcium intake in 1- to 11-year-old children: the Second National Health and Nutrition Examination Survey, 1976 to 1980. Pediatrics 1986;78:257–62.

[99] Blake KC, Mann M. Effect of calcium and phosphorus on the gastrointestinal absorption of 203Pb in man. Environ Res 1983;30:188–94.

[100] Heard MJ, Chamberlain AC. Uptake of Pb by human skeleton and comparative metabolism of Pb and alkaline earth elements. Health Phys 1984;47:857–65.

[101] Sargent JD, Dalton MA, O'Connor GT, et al. Randomized trial of calcium glycerophosphate-supplemented infant formula to prevent lead absorption. Am J Clin Nutr 1999;69:1224–30.

[102] Ettinger AS, Tellez-Rojo MM, Amarasiriwardena C, et al. Influence of maternal bone lead burden and calcium intake on levels of lead in breast milk over the course of lactation. Am J Epidemiol 2006;163(1):48–56.

[103] Goyer RA. Toxic and essential metal interactions. Annu Rev Nutr 1997;17:37–50.

[104] Ballew C, Bowman B. Recommending calcium to reduce lead toxicity in children: a critical review. Nutr Rev 2001;59:71–9.

[105] Bogden JD, Louria DB, Oleske JM. Regarding dietary calcium to reduce lead toxicity. Nutr Rev 2001;59:307–8.

[106] Yasui M, Ota K, Garruto RM. Effects of calcium-deficient diets on manganese deposition in the central nervous system and bones of rats. Neurotoxicology 1995;16:511–7.

[107] Murphy VA, Rosenberg JM, Smith QR, et al. Elevation of brain manganese in calcium-deficient rats. Neurotoxicology 1991;12:255–63.

[108] Felley-Bosco E, Diezi J. Dietary calcium restriction enhances cadmium-induced metallothionein synthesis in rats. Toxicol Lett 1992;60:139–44.

[109] Ravi K, Paliwal VK, Nath R. Induction of Cd-metallothionein in cadmium exposed monkeys under different nutritional stresses. Toxicol Lett 1984;22:21–6.

[110] Murphy VA, Embrey EC, Rosenberg JM, et al. Calcium deficiency enhances cadmium accumulation in the central nervous system. Brain Res 1991;557:280–4.

[111] Wang C, Brown S, Bhattacharyya MH. Effect of cadmium on bone calcium and 45Ca in mouse dams on a calcium-deficient diet: evidence of Itai-Itai-like syndrome. Toxicol Appl Pharmacol 1994;127:320–30.

[112] Sari MM, Blanusa M, Piasek M, et al. Effect of dietary calcium on cadmium absorption and retention in suckling rats. Biometals 2002;15:175–82.

[113] Walter A, Rimbach G, Most E, et al. Effects of calcium supplements to a maize-soya diet on the bioavailability of minerals and trace elements and the accumulation of heavy metals in growing rats. Journal of Veterinary Medicine–Series A 2000;47:367–77.

[114] Barton JC, Conrad ME, Nuby S, et al. Effects of iron on the absorption and retention of lead. J Lab Clin Med 1978;92:536–47.

[115] Hammad TA, Sexton M, Langenberg P. Relationship between blood lead and dietary iron intake in preschool children. A cross-sectional study. Ann Epidemiol 1996;6:30–3.

[116] Wright RO, Shannon MW, Wright RJ, et al. Association between iron deficiency and low-level lead poisoning in an urban primary care clinic. Am J Public Health 1999;89:1049–53.

[117] Wright RO, Tsaih SW, Schwartz J, et al. Association between iron deficiency and blood lead level in a longitudinal analysis of children followed in an urban primary care clinic. J Pediatr 2003;142:9–14.

[118] Cheng Y, Willett WC, Schwartz J, et al. Relation of nutrition to bone lead and blood lead levels in middle-aged to elderly men. The Normative Aging Study. Am J Epidemiol 1998; 147:1162–74.

[119] Chandra SV, Shukla GS. Role of iron deficiency in inducing susceptibility to manganese toxicity. Arch Toxicol 1976;35:319–23.

[120] Shukla A, Agarwal KN, Shukla GS. Effect of latent iron deficiency on the levels of iron, calcium, zinc, copper, manganese, cadmium and lead in liver, kidney and spleen of growing rats. Experientia 1990;46:751–2.

[121] Finley JW. Manganese absorption and retention by young women is associated with serum ferritin concentration. Am J Clin Nutr 1999;70:37–43.

[122] Groten JP, Luten JB, van Bladeren PJ. Dietary iron lowers the intestinal uptake of cadmium-metallothionein in rats. Eur J Pharmacol 1992;228:23–8.

[123] Flanagan PR, McLellan JS, Haist J, et al. Increased dietary cadmium absorption in mice and human subjects with iron deficiency. Gastroenterology 1978;74:841–6.

[124] Flanagan PR, Haist J, Valberg LS. Comparative effects of iron deficiency induced by bleeding and a low-iron diet on the intestinal absorptive interactions of iron, cobalt, manganese, zinc, lead and cadmium. J Nutr 1980;110:1754–63.

[125] Akesson A, Stal P, Vahter M. Phlebotomy increases cadmium uptake in hemochromatosis. Environ Health Perspect 2000;108:289–91.

[126] Zeng H, Uthus EO, Combs GF Jr. Mechanistic aspects of the interaction between selenium and arsenic. J Inorg Biochem 2005;99(6):1269–74.

[127] Rogan WJ, Dietrich KN, Ware JH, et al. Treatment of Lead-Exposed Children Trial Group. The effect of chelation therapy with succimer on neuropsychological development in children exposed to lead. N Engl J Med 2001;344:1421–6.

[128] Haynes E, Lanphear BP, Tohn E, et al. The effect of interior lead hazard controls on children's blood lead concentrations: a systematic evaluation. Environ Health Perspect 2002; 110(1):103–7.

[129] Weitzman M, Aschengrau A, Bellinger D, et al. Lead-contaminated soil abatement and urban children's blood lead levels. JAMA 1993;269(13):1647–54.

[130] Lanphear BP, Succop P, Roda S, et al. The effect of soil abatement on blood lead levels in children living near a former smelting and milling operation. Public Health Rep 2003; 118(2):83–91.

ELSEVIER
SAUNDERS

Pediatr Clin N Am
54 (2007) 177–203

PEDIATRIC CLINICS
OF NORTH AMERICA

Trends in Childhood Cancer Incidence: Review of Environmental Linkages

Irena Buka, MB, ChB, FRCPC[a,b,*], Samuel Koranteng, MB, ChB[a], Alvaro R. Osornio Vargas, MD, PhD[c]

[a]*Paediatric Environmental Health Specialty Unit, Misericordia Hospital, 3 West, 16940 – 87 Avenue, Edmonton, AB T5R 4H5, Canada*
[b]*Department of Paediatrics, University of Alberta, Edmonton, Alberta, Canada*
[c]*División de Investigación Básica, Instituto Nacional de Cancerología, Mexico City, Mexico*

Cancer in children is rare and accounts for about 1% of all malignancies. In the developed world, however, it is the commonest cause of disease-related deaths in childhood, carrying with it a great economic and emotional cost [1]. Declines in mortality for childhood cancers relate to improved survival with current treatment modalities [2,3].

In the United States each year 150 of every 1 million children under the age of 20 years are diagnosed with cancer, with a predominance in males [2]. In Europe, it is estimated that 157 per million children under the age of 20 years develop cancer annually, males predominantly [3]. Higher cancer rates occur in children younger than 5 years of age and again in children aged 15 to 19 years, with rates for 5- to 9-year-olds and 10- to 14-year-olds being fairly similar and lower [2]. The commonest malignancies are leukemia, central nervous system (CNS) tumors, and lymphomas, accounting for approximately 57% of all cases in those less than 20 years of age in Europe [3] and for 62.6% of cases in the same age cohort in the United States [2]. Gender and age trends may vary for specific cancers (eg, in Hodgkin's disease [HD], males predominate in those diagnosed under 15 years of age but females predominate in the 15- to 19-year-old age groups [2]).

Concern has been raised in the United States and Europe that overall rates of childhood cancer have been increasing since the 1970s [2–6]. The study of environmental links with respect to cancer has increased during

---

* Corresponding author. Paediatric Environmental Health Specialty Unit, Misericordia Community Hospital, 3 West, 16940 – 87 Avenue, Edmonton, AB T5R 4H5, Canada.
E-mail address: ibuka@cha.ab.ca (I. Buka).

0031-3955/07/$ - see front matter © 2007 Elsevier Inc. All rights reserved.
doi:10.1016/j.pcl.2006.11.010
pediatric.theclinics.com

178 BUKA et al

the same time period. In vitro studies have demonstrated radiation-induced chromosomal aberrations and mutations in peripheral blood lymphocytes [7,8]. Reports of body burdens of chemicals highlight children's exposures to carcinogens [9]. The study of trends in incidence may be a clue to identifying environmental links.

Linet and colleagues [10] reported a modest rise in the incidence of childhood leukemia resulting from an abrupt increase from 1983 to 1984, although 1989 rates declined. For CNS tumors, rates rose between 1983 and 1986 with statistical significance. Rates for certain skin cancers rose significantly, but the incidence of HD decreased modestly (Fig. 1).

Studies of temporal trends in the incidence of childhood leukemia have been inconsistent. An average annual 0.7% increased incidence of acute lymphoblastic leukemia (ALL) ($P = .005$) was reported by McNally and colleagues [11] from the Manchester Children's Tumor Registry in the United Kingdom from 1954 to 1998. Magnani and colleagues [12] reported a 2.6% annual increase in the incidence rate of ALL in the 1- to 4-year-old age group (95% confidence interval [CI], 1.13–4.13) in Piedmont Northwest Italy between 1975 and 1998. Hjalgrin and colleagues [13], however, found stable rates of leukemia in Nordic countries (Sweden, Denmark, Norway,

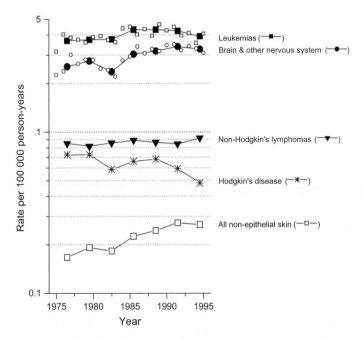

Fig. 1. Incidence of various childhood cancers, 1975–1995. (*Adapted from* Linet MS, Ries LAG, Smith MA, et al. Cancer Surveillance Series: recent trends in childhood cancer incidence and mortality in the United States. J Natl Cancer Inst 1999;91(12):1052; with permission of Oxford University Press.)

Finland, and Iceland). Clavel and colleagues [14] found no increased incidence in childhood leukemia in France between 1990 and 1999. McNally and colleagues [15] reported a 0.9% annual increase in incidence of childhood solid tumors in the Northwest of England between 1954 and 1998. Although these trends in part are recognized to be the result of improved diagnosis and reporting methods, investigators in some regions have found upward trends in certain childhood cancers.

Racial differences have been found for various malignancies, particularly for leukemia; in the United States the rate of leukemia was 41.6 per million for white children and was 25.8 per million for black children [2]. Incidence rates for childhood cancer in general were much lower in American Indians than in any other group in the United States [2]. The incidence of childhood leukemia in Costa Rica was described as being the highest in the world between 1981 and 1996 [16], with an overall age-standardized incidence rate of 56 per million person-years. McKinney and colleagues [5] described a higher incidence of all childhood cancers in South Asian children (of Indian, Pakistani, and Bangladeshi extraction) in Bradford, United Kingdom than in non-South Asian children, with significantly higher rates of acute myeloid leukemia (AML) in South Asian children. Scientists now are asking whether certain races bear genetic polymorphisms predisposing them to various childhood cancers or whether certain groups of children by their unique exposures are more vulnerable to specific childhood cancer.

Cancers are assumed to be multivariate, multifactorial diseases that occur when a complex and prolonged process involving genetic and environmental factors interact in a multistage sequence. This article explores the available evidence for this process, primarily from the environmental linkages perspective but including some evidence of the genetic factors. The first recognized environmental link with childhood cancer is believed to be Potts' published observation in 1775 of scrotal cancer occurring through exposure to soot in child chimney sweeps [7]. In the last few decades environmental linkages have been actively sought and described, but the evidence for causal association is still in the preliminary stages.

Radiation

The carcinogenic effects resulting from exposure to ionizing and non-ionizing radiation during the preconception, prenatal, and postnatal periods have been widely studied. Depending on the latency period, radiation-induced cancers may present during childhood or several decades after exposure.

High-dose ionizing radiation

Exposure to high-dose ionizing radiation leading to cancer has occurred in children after the atomic bombing at Hiroshima and Nagasaki in 1945

[17], the Chernobyl nuclear accident in Ukraine in 1986 [18–20], and following radiotherapy for childhood cancer [21–23] and tinea capitis [24]. Excess risk of leukemia has not been reported among children who were exposed in utero to radiation from the atomic bomb [17]. Nonetheless, children exposed postnatally at a younger age have been shown to have an increased risk of leukemia later in life (excess absolute risks of 0.6, 1.1, and 0.9 cases per 10 [4] person-years Sievert for ALL, AML, and CML, respectively) [25]. There is no current evidence to suggest an increased risk of leukemia among second- and third-generation offspring of atomic bomb-survivors in Japan [26].

Epidemiologic studies consistently have shown an elevated risk of radiation-induced thyroid cancer among children exposed to radionuclides especially iodine-131 (^{131}I) in Ukraine, Belarus, and Russia after the Chernobyl nuclear accident in Ukraine in 1986 (odds ratio [OR] at 1 Gy, 8.4; 95% CI, 4.1–17.3, compared with no exposure) [18–20,27]. Studies have clearly demonstrated an inverse relationship between the age at radiation exposure and the risk and severity of radiation-induced thyroid cancer [18,20] and also have documented a dose–response trend [19]. Although iodine supplementation has been shown to reduce the risk of ^{131}I-associated thyroid cancer in children (relative risk [RR], 0.34; 95% CI, 0.1–0.9), iodine deficiency tends to increase the risk (RR, 3.2; 95% CI, 1.9–5.5) [19]. The evidence linking childhood leukemia to radiation from the Chernobyl nuclear accident remains inconclusive, however [27].

Low-dose ionizing radiation

Children may be exposed to low-dose ionizing radiation during preconception, prenatal, and postnatal periods from fallouts from nuclear tests, residential proximity to nuclear facilities, parental occupational exposures to ionizing radiation, diagnostic radiographs, and residential exposure to radon decay products.

Nuclear weapons fallout

Excess relative risks of thyroid neoplasms (benign and malignant) have been observed among children exposed to fallouts from nuclear weapon testing in the United States and Russia [28,29]. The evidence linking childhood leukemia and atmospheric nuclear weapon testing has been less convincing [30].

Residential proximity to nuclear facilities

Reports from several countries indicate increased incidence of childhood cancer (eg, 5.0% total excess incidence, $P < .04$, in the United States) [31–34] and mortality rates [31–33] for children and young adults residing near nuclear facilities, although some studies have reported otherwise [34–37].

Studies have found excess local childhood cancer incidence and mortality rates compared with control populations or national averages [31,32,34,35]. The result from an extensive study in the United States suggests that radioactive emissions may account for one in nine childhood cancers among children less than 10 years old who live within 48 km of a nuclear facility in the United States [31]. There is evidence suggesting that children exposed to radiation from nuclear facilities at a younger age might be more susceptible to their leukemogenic effects [31,32]. Studies that have compared cancer incidence and mortality rates among children living in the vicinity of nuclear facilities before or during operation of such facilities and after shutdowns have failed to establish a clear risk pattern. Although in 1987 Magano and colleagues [38] found a reduction in cancer incidence in children less than 5 years of age following the shutdown of eight nuclear plants in the United States (a 25.0% reduction in nuclear counties compared with a 0.5% total reduction for other counties in the state; $P < .006$), Boice and colleagues [36,37] observed higher relative rates of childhood cancer and childhood leukemia mortality but lower rates of brain and other nervous tissue cancer before the operation of a nuclear facility in St. Lucie, Florida than after operation began. In Pennsylvania, however, they found a higher relative risk for childhood leukemia mortality before plant start-up than during operations or after closure (RR, 1.02, 0.81, 0.57, respectively) [37]. Other malignancies such as multiple myeloma and non-Hodgkin's lymphoma (NHL) have been associated with residential proximity to nuclear facilities in persons aged 0 to 24 years [34,35].

Residential exposure to radon

Radon and its decay products contribute significantly to the dose of natural and man-made ionizing radiation to which humans are exposed [39]. It is thought that radiation from radon and its decay products is delivered predominantly to the respiratory tract with minimal dose to other organs of the body, including the bone marrow [39]. Although residential exposure to radon has been found to increase the risk of lung cancer in adults moderately (excess OR, 0.14 per 100 Bqm^{-3}; 95% CI, −0.3–0.55 for a 5- to 35-year exposure) [40–42], studies have failed to demonstrate a consistent association between indoor radon levels and nonrespiratory cancers in both adults and children [43]. Some ecologic studies have reported an increased risk of ALL among children living in areas with high levels of indoor or ground levels of radon (RR, 5.67; 95% CI, 1.06–42.27) [44]; others have found a weak ecologic association between indoor radon and AML but not ALL [45]. Case-control studies also have shown a weak or no association between residential radon levels and AML or ALL in children [46–49]. One study in North Carolina reported increased childhood cancer mortality rates among children who resided in counties with higher ground-water radon concentrations (RR, 1.23; 95% CI, 1.11–1.37) [50].

Parental occupational exposures to ionizing radiations

Gardner's [51,52] hypothesis indicating that paternal exposure to ionizing radiation before conception may cause childhood leukemia and NHL has not been substantiated by other studies [53–56]. Although Drapper and colleagues [53] found a significantly elevated risk of childhood leukemia and NHL among children of men and women who were occupationally exposed to ionizing radiation before conception, no dose–response trend was observed. Although some have attributed the absence of a dose–response trend to other factors, such as an infectious agent spread through population mixing [53,56], others have hypothesized that exposure to a higher internal dose of radioisotopes among radiation workers may be responsible [57].

Diagnostic radiographs

Fetal irradiation (radiation doses in the order of the 10 mGy) resulting from prenatal exposure to diagnostic radiographs has been estimated to increase the risk of childhood cancer by approximately 6% per Gy [58]. In addition, increases in the number of X-ray exposures during the third trimester have been associated with increasing relative risks of childhood cancer (0.194 excess RR per film; 95% CI, 0.134–0.280). Results from other studies, including those that have evaluated the effects of in utero exposure to the atomic bomb in Japan, have not supported this association [15,53,59–62]. There is no consistent evidence to indicate that paternal preconception and early childhood exposure to diagnostic X-rays may significantly increase the risk of childhood cancer or childhood leukemia [53,59,60,62].

Non-ionizing radiation

There have been concerns about the carcinogenic effects of non-ionizing radiation in humans. Several studies have focused on the potential role of non-ionizing radiation such as UV radiation and extremely low-frequency electromagnetic field (ELF-EMF) in the development of childhood cancers.

Solar UV radiation

A large number of studies have examined the risk of developing melanoma and nonmelanoma skin cancers in adults after childhood exposure to solar UV radiation [63]. Evidence from ecologic studies suggests that the risk of both melanoma and nonmelanoma skin cancer may increase with increasing duration of residence in a high solar radiation environment, especially if exposure began at an early age [63,64]. There are limited data on the association between solar UV radiation and pediatric melanoma and nonmelanoma skin cancers, but a recent study in the United States demonstrated an elevated risk of pediatric melanoma among children exposed to higher levels of solar UV radiation (19% per kJ; 95% CI, 9–30) [65].

Extremely low-frequency electromagnetic fields

Children may be exposed to ELF-EMF (frequency range of 3–3000 Hz) during the preconception, prenatal, or postnatal periods [66]. Exposures during preconception and prenatal periods may result from parental exposures during these periods. Postnatal exposures may occur at home, day care, or school (because of residential or school proximity to power lines, electrical wiring, or use of electrical appliances) [67,68]. Although fewer studies have used personal monitoring devices to determine exposure to ELF in children [69,70], several other studies have used various surrogate indicators of exposure to ELF-EMF such as residential proximity to power lines [71–76], wire code category [69,70], and time-weighted average residential magnetic field levels [72]. The risk of childhood cancer, particularly leukemia and brain tumors, following paternal occupational exposure to ELF-EMF before conception [66,77], as well as the risk of prenatal [66,76–78] and early childhood exposures [72,79,80] to ELF-EMF, has been studied widely. The evidence linking ELF-EMF and childhood cancers remains inconclusive. In Canada, Green and colleagues [69,70] observed an increased risk of ALL only among children who were diagnosed with ALL before 6 years of age correlated with increasing personal exposure and time-weighted averages of magnetic fields within the outside perimeter of their residences (OR for $\mu T \geq 0.15$, 3.45; 95% CI, 1.14–10.45). No association was observed between childhood leukemia and residential proximity to power lines or personal exposures to electric fields [69,70]. Although a few studies have reported a link between childhood leukemia and residential proximity to power lines [71,74,81], a large number of case-control studies have failed to establish such an association [69,70,73,75,76]. There is insufficient evidence to support an association between paternal occupational exposure to ELF-EMF before conception and childhood leukemia and brain tumors [66,77]. A case-control study that used individual estimates of maternal occupational exposure to ELF-EMF found an increased risk of childhood leukemia among children whose mothers were exposed to the highest ($\geq 0.4 \mu T$) levels of ELF-EMF (OR, 2.5; 95% CI, 1.2–5.0) [78]. There is little or no evidence that exposure to ELF-EMF from electrical appliances such as infant incubators, electric blankets, and heated waterbeds is associated with childhood cancer [79,80].

Infectious etiology

Viral agents

The evidence supporting an infectious etiology of cancer in humans has been derived largely from the causal link between certain viruses and cancers in both children [82,83] and adults [84]. Hepatitis B virus (HBV) has been linked consistently to hepatocellular carcinoma (HCC) in children residing in areas hyperendemic for HBV infection [82,83]. Studies have consistently associated hepatitis B vaccination during early childhood with a decline in HCC incidence [83,85]. One study identified HBV genotype b as the predominant genotype associated with childhood HCC in Taiwan [82]. Recent data indicate that aflatoxin B1 (AFB_1), a potent mycotoxin and genotoxin, may interact synergistically with chronic HBV infection to increase the risk of HCC in both children [86] and adults (RR, 3.5; 95% CI; 1.5–8.1 for male adults) [87]. Higher levels of AFB_1-albumin adducts, a marker of AFB_1 exposure, have been detected in hepatitis B surface antigen (HBsAg)-positive children compared with HbsAg-negative children [86].

There is compelling evidence that Epstein-Barr virus (EBV) infection is associated with the development of HD in both children [88–91] and adults [84,89]. EBV genomes and membrane protein have been identified in Hodgkin and Reed-Sternberg cells in some cases of HD at a higher frequency in developing countries than in developed countries [88,89,92–94]. Nevertheless, available data suggest that EBV infection at an early age may play a significant role in the development of childhood HD in both developed [95,96] and developing countries [88,89,91,97]. Moreover, EBV infection has been linked to NHL, especially Burkitt's lymphoma, in children residing in the tropics [98,99]. Additionally, there is suggestive evidence indicating that repeated episodes of acute falciparum malaria may predispose children residing in the tropics to the development of Burkitt's lymphoma, possibly through reactivation of EBV-infected B lymphocytes [98,100].

Human herpesvirus 8 (HHS-8) is an established causal agent in all forms of Kaposi's sarcoma (KS), including AIDS-associated KS [86]. A higher prevalence of HHS-8 infection has been reported in HIV-1–positive than in HIV-1–negative children [101,102]. In developed countries, the estimated prevalence of HIV-associated malignancies in vertically infected children ranges from 1.8% to 5% [103–105]. In addition to KS, a high prevalence of NHL, particularly Burkitt's lymphoma, has been reported consistently among HIV-positive children [103–106]. KS or NHL may be the presenting illness in children infected with HIV, and both malignancies have been consequently classified as "AIDS-indicator diseases" [104].

Infectious etiology hypothesis for childhood leukemia

Socioeconomic and seasonal variations in the incidence of childhood leukemia [107–109] as well as the clustering of cases of childhood leukemia [110–112] suggest that infection may play a role in its development. Greaves [113] hypothesized that the precursor B-cell subtypes of ALL result from two independent mutations, the first occurring in utero or shortly after birth, and the second occurring later (coinciding with the age of peak incidence) with subsequent onset of overt childhood leukemia. Kinlen [111,114,115] proposed that childhood leukemia is a rare response to a common infection and that, in a relatively isolated community unexposed to such an infection, a rapid influx of newcomers would lead to an increased incidence of childhood leukemia. Both Greaves [113] and Kinlen [114,115] concluded that a delay in exposure to infection might result in an elevated risk of childhood leukemia. According to Smith's [116] hypothesis, childhood ALL in socioeconomically developed countries is caused by in utero exposure to infections. In keeping with Greave's [113] and Smith's [116] hypotheses, leukemic cells have been detected on Guthrie cards (newborn genetic screening cards) in children who later were diagnosed with B-precursor acute lymphoblastic leukemia [117].

The association between childhood leukemia and various surrogates of infection, including day care attendance [118–120]; breastfeeding [121], birth order [118,122,123], population mixing [110,124], socioeconomic status [107,125], and parental occupational contact levels [126,127], have been widely studied but with inconsistent results. Nevertheless, in a meta-analysis of studies on breastfeeding and the risk of childhood leukemia by Kwan and colleagues [121], both short-term ($\leq$ 6 months) and long-term ($\geq$ 6 months) breastfeeding was found to be significantly associated with a reduced risk of childhood ALL and AML. A review of studies on the infectious etiology of childhood leukemia by McNally and Eden [128] found evidence suggestive of a protective effect of breast-feeding, summer peak incidence of childhood leukemia, and a predisposition to childhood leukemia caused by prenatal exposure to infections.

Air pollution

Traffic-related air pollution (mobile sources)

Diesel exhaust has been classified by the International Agency for Research on Cancer (IARC) as a "probable human carcinogen" [129]. Various organic constituents of diesel exhaust particles, including benzene and polycyclic aromatic hydrocarbons, have shown mutagenic and/or chromosomal aberration effects in bacteria, animals and human cells [130–132]. Prenatal exposure to airborne polycyclic aromatic hydrocarbons has been associated with chromosomal aberrations in cord blood lymphocytes [133]. In vitro studies also have demonstrated the carcinogenic potential of gasoline exhaust particles [129,132]. Epidemiologic studies have used various measures of exposure to vehicle exhaust during the prenatal period or early childhood to investigate the role of vehicle exhaust in the development of pediatric malignancies. These include measures residential traffic density [134–136], distance-weighted traffic density [137], residential proximity to main roads [138,139], and estimated residential levels of indicators of traffic-related air pollution (eg, benzene, and nitric oxide [NO_2]) [139–142]. Three studies have reported a negative association between childhood leukemia and residential traffic density [134,136,142], although Savitz and Feingold [135] found a significant association between childhood leukemia and residential traffic density. Another study in Italy that used information on traffic density, vehicles emissions, and weather conditions to estimate annual mean ambient benzene concentration reported an increased risk of childhood leukemia among children exposed to higher levels of benzene (estimated annual average of $> 10 \mu g^{-3}$ compared with $< 0.1 \mu g^{-3}$) from road traffic emissions (RR, 3.91; 95% CI, 1.36–11.27) [140]. Raaschou-Niesel and colleagues [142] demonstrated an elevated risk of HD but not childhood leukemia among children exposed in utero to higher residential concentrations of NO_2 and benzene estimated from road traffic emissions (25%, P for trend $= .06$, and 51%, P for trend $= .05$ for a doubling in concentrations of NO_2 and benzene, respectively). Ambient levels of NO_2 in Sweden also have been associated with CNS tumors in children but not with childhood leukemia [141]. Evidence from studies in Great Britain suggests that children who are exposed to 1, 3-butadiene and carbon monoxide, primarily derived from engine exhausts, during the prenatal or early childhood are more likely to develop childhood cancers, including childhood leukemia [143,144]. Moreover, excess relative risks for all childhood cancers have been reported among children living within 1.0 km of bus stations (RR, 3.14; 95% CI, 2.69–3.68), industrial transport centers (RR, 1.88; 95% CI, 1.62–2.16) and railways (RR, 1.62; 95% CI, 1.48–1.77) [143]. There is lack of epidemiologic evidence to support a link between childhood leukemia and residential proximity to main roads [139,141]. Given the limited number of studies, variations in study designs, and inconsistencies among study results, no firm conclusion can be made with respect to the link between vehicle exhaust and childhood cancer.

Industrial air pollution

In addition to traffic-related air pollution, air pollution from stationary sources has been associated with childhood cancer. Studies in the United Kingdom have documented excess relative risks for childhood cancer for children living within 0.3 km of hotspots for carbon monoxide, particulate matter size PM_{10}, nitrogen oxides, benzene, benzo(a)pyrene, 1,3-butadiene, dioxins, and volatile organic compounds [143,144]. Furthermore, residential proximity to potential sources of benzene, such as oil installations [143], gas stations, and automobile repair garages, during early childhood has been linked to childhood cancers, including childhood leukemia [139]. For example, Steffen and colleagues [139] observed a significant association between childhood acute nonlymphocytic leukemia and residential proximity to gas stations and automobile repair garages during early childhood (OR, 7.7; 95% CI, 1.7–34.3).

A large population-based study in California found significantly elevated risks of leukemia among children exposed to the highest level of 25 hazardous air pollutants from combined sources (mobile, smaller stationary, and point sources) (RR, 1.21; 95% CI, 1.03–1.42) as well as point sources (large industrial facilities) (RR, 1.32; 95% CI, 1.11–1.57) [145].

Environmental tobacco smoke

Although both active and passive tobacco smoking have been unequivocally linked to lung cancer in adults [146,147], studies in children, which have focused mainly on the link between active parental tobacco smoking or environmental tobacco smoke and childhood brain tumors [148–151], leukemia [152,153], and lymphoma [151], have been less consistent. A few studies have significantly linked paternal cigarette smoking before conception with childhood cancers, including neuroblastoma and lymphoma [151,154]. Several other studies, however, did not observe significant associations between childhood brain tumors (including neuroblastoma) and paternal smoking before pregnancy or active maternal smoking [148–150]. Filippini and colleagues [155] found an increased risk of CNS tumors in children resulting from active or passive maternal tobacco smoking during the first 5 weeks of pregnancy (OR, 1.5; 95% CI, 1.0–2.3) but not before conception. There is no strong epidemiologic evidence to suggest that paternal smoking before conception or prenatal exposure to environmental tobacco smoke will increase the risk of childhood leukemia [153,156] or germ cell tumors [157,158]. The results from studies that have examined the relationship between parental cigarette smoking and the risk of hepatoblastoma in children have been inconsistent [159,160]. Despite the inconsistencies among study results, mutagenicity and genotoxicity caused by transplacental exposure to environmental tobacco smoke have been well documented [161,162].

Medications, food, drugs

In the 1970s it was confirmed that intrauterine exposure to diethylstilboestrol predisposed young women to developing vaginal adenocarcinoma between the ages of 15 and 29 years. The eighth week of pregnancy, the time at which the female lower genital tract is developing, is thought to be the critical period for exposure to diethylstilboestrol [163].

The Children's Cancer Group studied parental use of medication during pregnancy in the mother and 1 year before pregnancy in both parents. Maternal use of vitamins (OR, 0.7; 99% CI, 0.5–1.0) and iron (OR, 0.5; 99% CI, 0.7–1.0) was found to decrease the risk of ALL. Maternal use of antihistamines and other allergic remedies was associated with infant ALL [164].

Food consumption by children in California under the age of 2 years was studied. Regular consumption of oranges, bananas, and orange juice was associated with a reduction in the risk of childhood leukemia. Ingestion of hot dogs and luncheon meats showed no association [165]. A previous study in California had shown an association between children's intake of hot dogs (OR, 9.5; 95% CI, 1.6–57.6 for 12 or more hot dogs per month; trend $P = .01$) as well as the father's intake of hot dogs (OR, 11.0; CI, 1.2–98.7 for highest intake category; trend $P = .01$) with some increase in risk of childhood leukemia. In this study fruit intake did not show any association with protection [166]. There has been interest in the study of drinking water contaminants and childhood leukemia. Postnatal exposures to trihalomethanes (OR, 1.54; 95% CI, 0.78–3.03), chloroform (OR, 1.63; 95% CI, 0.84–3.19) and zinc (OR, 2.48; 95% CI 0.99–6.24) were associated with increased risk [167]. A meta-analysis of maternal cured meat intake during pregnancy showed a summary relative risk of childhood brain tumors in the offspring (RR, 1.68; 95% CI, 1.30–2.17, a statistically significant increased risk) [168].

Amphetamines and mind-altering drugs used by both parents before and during the index pregnancy increased the risk of ALL in their children (OR, 2.8; 99% CI, 0.5–15.6 for amphetamines; OR, 1.8; 99% CI; 1.1–3.0 for mind-altering drugs) [164]. A case-controlled study of maternal marijuana use showed an association with ALL among the offspring [169]. A further case-controlled study showed that maternal use of marijuana and cocaine in the year before the child's birth increased the risk of rhabdomyosarcoma in the children threefold (95% CI, 1.4–6.5) and 5.1-fold (95% CI, 1.0–25.0), respectively [170]. Marijuana use in the father increased the risk twofold (95% CI, 1.3–3.3), and cocaine use increased the risk 2.1-fold (95% CI, 0.9–4.9) [170].

Scientific evidence suggesting dietary factors as well as parental medication and/or drug use may be contributing to the development of childhood cancer is inconsistent. Further investigation incorporating identification of susceptible individuals may provide relevant evidence.

Pesticides

Recent studies have supported an increased risk of childhood cancer (standardized incidence ratio, 1.36; 95% CI, 1.03–1.79), especially for all lymphomas (standardized incidence ratio, 2.18; 95% CI, 1.13–41.9), in offspring of parents working as pesticide applicators, particularly if chemically resistant gloves were not used [171]. Another study found a significantly increased risk of childhood leukemia (OR, 2.8; 95% CI, 1.4–5.7) if professional pest control services were used in the home for 1 year before and 3 years after birth of the child. The risk was highest when insecticide exposures, especially indoor exposures, occurred in pregnancy [172]. A national case-controlled study in Australia showed an excess of case mothers whose offspring developed Ewing's sarcoma if the mother worked on a farm at conception or during pregnancy (OR, 2.8; 95% CI, 0.5–12.0), and the risk doubled if she handled pesticides [173]. A study of astrocytoma and primitive neuroectodermal tumors in the United States and Canada, however, showed little indication for an association with cumulative and average parental exposures to pesticides [174]. A previous review of 31 studies examining occupational and residential exposures to pesticides by either parent or children showed a modest risk of developing several tumors, but conclusions could not be drawn because of methodologic limitations [175]. The methodology of assessing exposure to pesticides, in general, is particularly challenging and requires identifying accurate biomarkers.

Parental occupational exposures

For several decades researchers have been sought links between childhood cancer and chemical exposure through parental occupation during periconception, pregnancy, and childhood of their offspring. Recently, results from the United Kingdom Child Cancer Study examined parental occupation and related periconceptional exposures and failed to show strong evidence linking parental exposures with an increased risk of childhood cancer. A small significant increased risk for childhood leukemia was found to be associated with paternal occupational exposure to exhaust fumes, however (OR, 1.23; 95% CI, 1.00–1.52), inhaled particulate hydrocarbons (OR, 1.14; 95% CI, 0.90–1.45), and driving (OR, 1.14; 95% CI, 0.89–1.72) [54]. A pooled analysis of three German population-based case-control studies, using methodologies similar to those of a large United States study, showed results inconsistent with those of the United States study [176]. The German analyses found maternal exposure to paints or lacquers during the periconceptional period was related to an increased risk of ALL (OR, 1.6; 95% CI, 1.1–2.4) [176]. Maternal exposure during the index pregnancy was related to an increased risk of childhood ALL (OR, 2.0; 95% CI, 1.2–3.3), consistent with observations from the United States study, which also found an association with maternal exposure to solvents, not found in Quebec, Canada [177], and parental exposure to plastic materials, not confirmed by the German analysis [176]. In 2001, a seven-country case-controlled study found an increased risk of childhood brain tumors when fathers worked in agriculture (OR, 2.2; 95% CI, 1.0–4.7) [178]. De Roos and colleagues [179] reported an association between neuroblastoma and paternal exposures to hydrocarbons, lacquer thinner, turpentine, wood dust, and sawdust. Assessing chemical environmental links to childhood cancer through parental occupational exposure remains a methodologic challenge. Studies generally are performed by self-administered questionnaires with or without interviews. Possible exposures as well as timing of exposures are considered, but neither may be the optimal way of assessing exposures of relevance. Exposures can be assessed accurately only through regular prospective biomonitoring.

Cancer, genes, and the environment

Cancer is a multifactorial and multistage group of diseases in which gene alterations play a critical role [180]. In children, development and growth open multiple windows of opportunity for environmental factors to alter genetically controlled cellular processes that could lead to cancer. Therefore, risky exposures could occur as early as during pregnancy and manifest during childhood or later in life. It has long been known that some hereditary genetic alterations predispose children to cancer. In xeroderma pigmentosum, for example, gene repair is defective, and exposures to sunlight can trigger skin cancer in those individuals [181]. Most childhood cancers, however, are not the result of inherited predisposition but rather are assumed to be the results of randomly occurring processes, in which individual susceptibility plays a major role [182]. Increasing exposures to environmental factors begs the question of how much "randomness" and "susceptibility" are the result of chemical and physical challenges imposed by exposure to toxicants in the environment. Pesticides, radiation, and air pollution are examples of common factors to which children may be exposed on a daily basis, promoting gene–environment interactions. Gene–environment interactions may result in health effects as a consequence of induced alterations or naturally occurring polymorphisms in genes that mediate gene repair or in genes that mediate toxicants or xenobiotics metabolism.

Environmental exposures of parents can result in gene alterations that may lead to childhood cancer. Increased maternal dietary intake of bioflavonoids may increase the risk of AML tenfold. Bioflavonoids can induce DNA breaks at specific sites relevant to AML (MLL gene), which is probably mediated by topoisomerase II inhibition [183,184]. In neuroblastoma, loss of heterozygosity of the short arm of chromosome one is described; the cause of this mutation as yet is unknown [2].

Naturally occurring genetic polymorphisms could explain genetic susceptibility to specific environmental challenges. The study of ALL and polymorphisms of various genes involved in bioactivation and detoxification of xenobiotics has shown that combinations of polymorphisms represent risk-elevating genotypes. Deletions or sequence alterations in genes that encode for enzymes involved in detoxification (glutathione S-transferase, cytochromes [P-450, CYP]) or bioactivation (N-acetyltransferases) result in those polymorphisms linked to increased risk for ALL in children (OR, 1.5–10.3) [185–187]. Another example is the linkage between the genetic polymorphism that prevents paraoxonase detoxifying pesticide activity and increases the risk for children to develop primitive neuroectodermal tumors in the brain (OR ~ 2.5) [188].

Current research using new gene and statistical methodologies promote optimism about future understanding of cancer–gene–environment interactions.

Childhood environmental exposures and adult cancers

Early exposure to environmental carcinogens may lead to childhood cancer or adult-onset malignancies, depending on the latency period of the particular cancer involved [19,189,190]. Although no significantly higher incidence of adult malignancies has been observed among children exposed in utero to radiation from the 1945 atomic bomb in Japan, an excess risk of breast cancer, basal cell carcinoma, and nervous system tumors have been reported among adults exposed at an early age ($<$ 20 years) [189–194]. There is no reported increased risk of thyroid cancer, leukemia, or other malignancies in adults exposed at an early age to radionuclides (^{131}I) from the Chernobyl nuclear disaster [27].

Thyroid carcinoma, breast cancer, and other secondary malignancies have developed in adults several decades after radiotherapy for childhood primary malignancies [21,22,195]. Children who had radiotherapy for tinea capitis are known to have an elevated risk of developing malignant brain tumors (0.47 excess absolute risk per Gy per 10^4 person-years; 95% CI, 0.12–0.53) and basal cell carcinoma of the head and neck region (RR, 3.6; 95% CI, 2.3–5.9) [24,196].

Chemotherapy (alkylating agents, anthracyclines, and topoisomerase II inhibitors) for various childhood primary cancers may predispose to various types of secondary adult-onset malignancies (eg, leukemia and bone cancer), depending on the particular medication used and the type of primary cancer involved [197]. Prenatal exposure to diethylstilboestrol is a known risk factor for clear cell adenocarcinoma of the vagina in young women [163].

There is evidence that early residential exposure to high levels of solar UV radiation and childhood sunburns may significantly increase the risk of developing cutaneous malignant melanoma (CMM) later in life (OR for superficial spreading melanoma, 1.8; 95% CI, 1.1–2.8 for sunburn episodes before age 15 years) [64,198]. Moreover, exposure to artificial UV radiation from indoor tanning devices during adolescence has been identified as a risk factor for CMM in adulthood [199]. It is not clear whether childhood exposure to solar radiation confers a greater risk of CMM than exposure in adulthood [200,201].

Controversy exists with respect to childhood exposure to environmental tobacco smoke and the risk of breast cancer, lung cancer, leukemia, and lymphoma in adults [151,202–206]. Childhood exposure to domestic wood smoke as well as the ingestion of food containing nitrosamines (salted fish and other preserved food) has been associated with the development of adult-onset nasopharyngeal carcinoma in Southern China and Southern Asia [207]. Although aflatoxin B1 is known to interact synergistically with HBV in the development of HCC, and aflatoxin M1, a metabolite of aflatoxin B1 has been detected in human milk, it is not known how early-life exposure to this mycotoxin would influence the risk of developing adult HCC [87,208,209].

HHS-8 has been linked causally to all types of KS [83], and HBV has been associated with HCC in children and adults [82,83,87]. EBV infection is a risk factor for HD and nasopharyngeal carcinoma [83,86,210]. A higher prevalence of KS and Hodgkin's lymphoma has been observed among children vertically infected with HIV [102–105]. The impact of prenatal and early childhood exposures to these viruses on the risk of their respective adult-onset cancers remains unclear.

Table 1
Environmental linkages for childhood cancer

Environmental factor	Level of evidence	Type of cancer (exposure)
High-dose ionizing radiation	Conclusive evidence[a]	Thyroid cancer (Chernobyl nuclear disaster)
	Compelling evidence[b]	Childhood cancer (Hiroshima atom bomb)
	Inconclusive evidence[c]	Childhood leukemia (Chernobyl nuclear disaster and Hiroshima atom bomb)
	Some evidence[d]	Childhood cancer (radiotherapy)
Nuclear weapon fallout	Compelling evidence	Thyroid neoplasms (benign and malignant)
	Some evidence	Childhood leukemia
Residential proximity to nuclear facilities	Inconclusive evidence	Childhood cancer, childhood leukemia, multiple myeloma, NHL
Residential exposure to radon	Some evidence	Childhood leukemia
Parental occupational exposures to ionizing radiations	Some evidence	Childhood leukemia, NHL
Diagnostic radiographs	Compelling evidence	Childhood cancer (fetal exposure)
Solar UV radiation	Some evidence	Pediatric melanoma
ELF-EMF	Inconclusive evidence	ALL, brain tumors
Viral agents	Compelling evidence	HCC (HBV)
	Compelling evidence	HD, NHL, BL (EBV)
	Compelling evidence	KS (HHS-8)
	Compelling evidence	KS, NHL, BL (HIV)
Infective hypothesis	Some evidence	Childhood leukemia (prenatal exposure to infections, breastfeeding protection
Traffic-related air pollution	Inconclusive evidence	Childhood cancers, childhood leukemia, HD
Industrial air pollution	Compelling evidence	Childhood cancer, childhood leukemia
Environmental tobacco smoke	Inconclusive evidence	Brain tumors, childhood leukemia, lymphoma, germ cell tumors, hepatoblastoma
Medications, food, drugs	Conclusive evidence	Vaginal adenocarcinoma (prenatal diethylstilboestrol)
	Inconclusive evidence	ALL, Brain tumors (hot dogs, lunch meat)
	Inconclusive evidence	Childhood leukemia (fruit intake – protective)
	Some evidence	ALL (maternal antihistamines, maternal vitamins and iron – protective)
	Some evidence	ALL, Rhabdomyosarcoma (maternal/paternal marijuana, amphetamines)

(continued on next page)

Table 1 (*continued*)

Environmental factor	Level of evidence	Type of cancer (exposure)
Pesticides	Some evidence	Childhood cancer, childhood leukemia, lymphomas, CNS tumors
Parental occupational exposures Childhood exposure leading to adult cancers	Inconclusive evidence	ALL, brain tumors, Neuroblastomas
High-dose ionizing radiation	Compelling evidence	Thyroid carcinoma, breast cancer, bone cancer, malignant brain tumors, basal cell carcinomas of head and neck (radiotherapy) breast cancer, leukemia, nervous system tumor (atomic bomb)
	Inconclusive evidence	Thyroid cancers, leukemias (Chernobyl nuclear disaster)
Residential proximity to nuclear facilities	Inconclusive evidence	Childhood cancer, childhood leukemia, multiple myeloma, NHL
Residential exposure to radon	Some evidence	Lung cancer
Solar UV radiation	Compelling evidence	All skin cancers
Environmental tobacco smoke	Conclusive evidence	Lung cancer

Abbreviations: ALL, acute lymphoblastic leukemia; BL, Burkitt's lymphoma; CNS, central nervous system; EBV, Epstein-Barr virus; ELF-EMF, extremely low-frequency electromagnetic field; HBV, hepatitis B virus; HCC, hepatocellular carcinoma; HD, Hodgkin's disease; HHS-8, human herpesvirus 8; KS, Kaposi's sarcoma; NHL, non-Hodgkin's lymphoma.

[a] Conclusive evidence: cause and effect are undoubtedly linked with evidence of a dose–response trend.

[b] Compelling evidence: although the data linking cause and effect is substantial, there is no consistent evidence of a dose- response trend and/or evidence confirming timing and dosing of exposure.

[c] Inconclusive evidence: extensive studies have produced inconsistent results.

[d] Some evidence: early evidence suggests links.

Summary

Although evidence linking environmental associations in the development of cancers is accumulating (Table 1), the answer to a parent's question, "Why did my child get cancer?" is still elusive. An environmental history may reveal a combination of possible exposures as outlined in this article. The question of "Why my child?" is, at this stage of knowledge, more difficult to answer. Progress in this area will continue if the questions are asked. Environmental history taking and closer investigation of observations regarding incidence trends and possible clusters of cases have provided answers in the past. Availability of reliable biomarkers to study environmental exposures accurately through dosing, timing, and windows of opportunity are key to evaluating etiologic circumstances of childhood cancer. Ongoing gene–environment study will bring clinicians closer to offering anticipatory, preventative advice, probably through identification of susceptible, exposed individuals.

Acknowledgments

The authors sincerely thank Bronia Heilik, BA, BLS, and Elizabeth Mortimer for library assistance, and Michelle Huculak for her administrative assistance.

References

[1] Ferlay J, Bray F, Pisani P, et al. GLOBOCAN 2000. Cancer incidence, mortality and prevalence worldwide, version 1.0. IARC CancerBase No. 5. Lyon (France): IARCPress; 2001.

[2] Ries LAG Smith MA, Gurney JG, et al, editors. Cancer incidence and survival among children and adolescents: United States SEER Program 1975–1995. Bethesda (MD): National Cancer Institute, SEER Program 1999. NIH Pub. No. 99–4649.

[3] Steliarova-Foucher E, Stiller C, Kaatsch P, et al. Geographical patterns and time trends of cancer incidence and survival among children and adolescents in Europe since the 1970s (the ACCIS project): an epidemiological study. Lancet 2004;364:2097–105.

[4] Dalmasso P, Pastore G, Zuccolo L, et al. Temporal trends in the incidence of childhood leukemia, lymphomas and solid tumors in north-west Italy, 1967–2001. A report of the Childhood Cancer Registry of Piedmont. Hematol J 2005;90(9):1197–204.

[5] McKinney PA, Feltbower RG, Parslow RC, et al. Patterns of childhood cancer by ethnic group in Bradford, UK 1974-1997. Eur J Cancer 2003;39:92–7.

[6] Dreifaldt AC, Carlberg M, Hardell L. Increasing incidence rates of childhood malignant diseases in Sweden during the period 1960–1998. Eur J Cancer 2004;40:1351–60.

[7] Gochfeld M. Chronologic history of occupational medicine. J Occup Environ Med 2005; 47(2):96–114.

[8] Kote-Jaria Z, Salmon A, Mengistu T, et al. Increased chromosomal damage after irradiation of lymphocytes from BRCA1 mutation carriers. Br J Cancer 2006;94(2):308–10.

[9] Third National Report on Human Exposure to Environmental Chemicals. NCEH pub. No. 05-0570. Atlanta (GA); 2005. p. 1–475. Available at: http://www.cdc.gov/exposurereport/3rd/pdf/thirdreport.pdf. Accessed February 15, 2006.

[10] Linet MS, Ries LAG, Smith MA, et al. Cancer surveillance series: recent trends in childhood cancer incidence and mortality in the United States. J Natl Cancer Inst 1999;91(12):1051–8.

[11] McNally RJQ, Cairns DP, Eden OB, et al. Examination of temporal trends in the incidence of childhood leukaemias and lymphomas provides aetiological clues. Leukemia 2001;15: 1612–8.

[12] Magnani C, Dalmasso P, Pastore G, et al. Increasing incidence of childhood leukemia in northwest Italy, 1975–98. Int J Cancer 2003;105:552–7.

[13] Hjalgrim LL, Rostgaard K, Schmiegelow K, et al. Age- and sex-specific incidence of childhood leukemia by immunophenotype in the Nordic countries. J Natl Cancer Inst 2003; 95(20):1539–44.

[14] Clavel J, Goubin A, Auclerc MF, et al. Incidence of childhood leukaemia and non-Hodgkin's lymphoma in France: national registry of childhood leukaemia and lymphoma, 1990–1999. Eur J Cancer Prev 2004;13:97–103.

[15] McNally RJQ, Kelsey AM, Cairns DP, et al. Temporal increases in the incidence of childhood solid tumors seen in northwest England (1954–1998) are likely to be real. Cancer 2001; 92(7):1967–76.

[16] Monge P, Wesseling C, Rodriguez AC, et al. Childhood leukaemia in Costa Rica, 1981–96. Paediatr Perinat Epidemiol 2002;16:210–8.

[17] Jablon S, Kato H. Childhood cancer in relation to prenatal exposure to atomic-bomb radiation. Lancet 1970;296(7681):1000–3.

[18] Tronko MD, Bogdanova TI, Komissarenko IV, et al. Thyroid carcinoma in children and adolescents in Ukraine after the Chernobyl nuclear accident. Cancer 1999;86:149–56.

[19] Cardis E, Kesminiene A, Ivanov V, et al. Risk of thyroid cancer after exposure to ^{131}I in childhood. J Natl Cancer Inst 2005;97:724–32.

[20] Farahati J, Demidchik EP, Biko J, et al. Inverse association between age at the time of radiation exposure and extent of disease in cases of radiation-induced childhood thyroid carcinoma in Belarus. Cancer 2000;88:1470–6.

[21] Sigvidson AJ, Ronkers CM, Mertens AC, et al. Primary thyroid cancer after a first tumour in children (the Childhood Cancer Survival Study): a nested case-control study. Lancet 2005;365:2014–23.

[22] Acharya S, Sarafoglou K, LaQuaglia M, et al. Thyroid neoplasms after therapeutic radiation for malignancies during childhood or adolescence. Cancer 2003;97:2397–403.

[23] Bhatia S, Robson LL, Oberlin O, et al. Breast cancer and other second neoplasms after childhood Hodgkin's disease. N Engl J Med 1996;334:745–51.

[24] Shore RL, Moseson M, Xue X, et al. Skin cancer after X-ray treatment for scalp ringworm. Radiat Res 2002;157:410–8.

[25] Preston DL, Kusumi S, Tomonaga M, et al. Cancer incidence in atomic bomb survivors. 3. Leukemia, lymphoma and multiple myelopma, 1950–1987. Radiat Res 1994;137(Suppl): S68–97.

[26] Kusuyama M, Matsumoto K, Matsumoto T, et al. Childhood leukemia: epidemiological investigation and effectiveness of treatment in Nagasaki over the past 12 years. Acta Paediatr Japonica 1997;39:181–7.

[27] Moysich KB, Menezes RJ, Michalek AM. Chernobyl-related ionizing radiation exposure and cancer risk: an epidemiological review. Lancet Oncol 2002;3(5):269–79.

[28] Kerber RA, Till JE, Simon SL, et al. A cohort study of thyroid disease in relation to fallout from nuclear weapons testing. JAMA 1993;270(17):2076–82.

[29] Lund E, Galanti MR. Incidence of thyroid cancer in Scandinavia following fallout from atomic bomb testing: an analysis of birth cohorts. Cancer Causes Control 1999;10(3):181–7.

[30] Darby SC, Olsen JH, Doll R, et al. Trends in childhood leukemia in Nordic countries in relation to fallout from atmospheric nuclear weapons testing. BMJ 1992;304(6833):1005–9.

[31] Magano JJ, Sherman J, Chang C, et al. Elevated childhood cancer incidence proximate to U.S. nuclear power plants. Arch Environ Health 2003;58(2):74–82.

[32] Guizard AV, Boutou O, Pottier D, et al. The incidence of childhood leukemia around the La Hague nuclear waste reprocessing plant (France): a survey for the years 1978–1998. J Epidemiol Community Health 2001;55:469–74.

[33] Goldsmith JR. Nuclear installations and childhood cancer in the UK: mortality and incidence for 0-9- year-old children, 1971–1980. Sci Total Environ 1992;127:13–35.

[34] Drapper GJ, Stiller CA, Cartwright RA, et al. Cancer in Cumbria and in the vicinity of the Sellafield nuclear installation, 1963–90. BMJ 1993;306(6870):89–94.

[35] Lopez-Abente G, Arogonies N, Pollan M, et al. Leukemia, lymphoma, and myeloma mortality in the vicinity of nuclear power plants and nuclear fuel facilities in Spain. Cancer Epidemiol Biomarkers Prev 1999;8:925–34.

[36] Boice JD, Mumma MT, Blot WJ, et al. Childhood cancer mortality in relation to St Lucie nuclear power station. J Radiol Prot 2005;25:229–40.

[37] Boice JD Jr, Bigbee WL, Mumma MT, et al. Cancer mortality in counties near two former nuclear materials processing facilities in Pennsylvania, 1950-1995. Health Phys 2003;85(6): 691–700.

[38] Magano JJ, Gould JM, Sternglass EJ, et al. Infant death and childhood cancer reductions after plant closings in the United States. Arch Environ Health 2002;57(1):23–31.

[39] Parker L, Craft AW. Radon and childhood cancers. Eur J Cancer 1996;32A(2):201–4.
[40] Darby S, Hill D, Auvinen J, et al. Radon in homes and risk of lung cancer: collaborative analysis of individual data from 13 European case-control studies. BMJ 2005; 330:223–7.
[41] Kreweski D, Lubin JH, Zielinski JM, et al. Residential radon and risk of lung cancer: a combines analysis of 7 North American case-control studies. Epidemiology 2005;16(2):137–45.
[42] Wichman HE, Rosario AS, Heid IM, et al. Increased lung cancer risk due to residential radon in a pooled and extended analysis of studies in Germany. Health Phys 2005;888(1): 71–9.
[43] Laurier D, Valenty M, Tirmarche M. Radon exposure and the risk of leukemia: a review of epidemiological studies. Health Phys 2001;81(3):271–88.
[44] Kohli S, Noorlind B, Lofman O. Childhood leukemia in areas with different radon levels; a spatial and temporal analysis using GIS. J Epidemiol Community Health 2000;54:822–6.
[45] Evrad AS, Hemon D, Billon S, et al. Ecological association between indoor radon concentration and childhood leukemia incidence in France, 1990-1998. Eur J Cancer Prev 2005;14: 147–57.
[46] Lubin JH, Linet MS, Boice JD, et al. Case-control study of childhood acute lymphoblastic leukemia and residential radon exposure. J Natl Cancer Inst 1998;90(4):294–300.
[47] UK Childhood Cancer Study Investigators. The United Kingdom childhood cancer study of exposure to domestic sources of ionizing radiation: 1; radon gas. Br J Cancer 2002;86: 1721–6.
[48] Axelson O, Fredrikson M, Akerblom G, et al. Leukemia in childhood and adolescence and exposure to ionizing radiation in homes built from uranium-containing alum shale concrete. Epidemiology 2002;13:146–50.
[49] Steinbuch M, Weinberg CR, Buckley JD, et al. Indoor residential radon exposure and risk of childhood acute myeloid leukemia. Br J Cancer 1999;81(5):900–6.
[50] Collman GW, Loomis DP, Sandler DP. Childhood cancer mortality and radon concentration in drinking water in North Carolina. Br J Cancer 1991;63:626–9.
[51] Gardner MJ, Snee MP, Hall AJ, et al. Results of case-control study of leukemia and lymphoma among young people near Sellafield nuclear plant in West Cumbria. BMJ 1990;300: 423–9.
[52] Gardner MJ. Paternal occupations of children with leukeumia. BMJ 1992;305:715.
[53] Drapper GJ, Little MP, Soharan T, et al. Cancer in the offspring of radiation workers: a record linkage study. BMJ 1997;315:1181–8.
[54] McKinney PA, Fear NT, Stockton D. Parental occupation at periconception: findings from the United Kingdom Childhood Cancer Study. Occup Environ Med 2003;60:901–9.
[55] Roman E, Doyle P, Maconochie N, et al. Cancer in children of nuclear industry employees: report on children aged under 25 years from nuclear industry family study. BMJ 1999; 318(7196):1443–50.
[56] Sorahan T, Haylock RG, Muirhead CR, et al. Cancer in the offspring of radiation workers: an investigation of employment timing and a reanalysis using updated dose information. Br J Cancer 2003;89(7):1215–20.
[57] Busby C, Cato MS. Cancer in the offspring of radiation workers: exposure to internal radiation may be responsible. BMJ 1998;316:1672.
[58] Doll R, Wakeford R. Risk of childhood cancer from fetal irradiation. Br J Radiol 1997;70: 130–9.
[59] Patton T, Olshan AF, Neglia JP, et al. Parental exposure to medical radiation and neuroblastoma in offspring. Paediatr Perinat Epidemiol 2004;18:178–85.
[60] Shu XO, Potter JD, Linet M, et al. Diagnostic X-rays and ultrasound and risk of childhood acute lymphoblastic leukemia by immunophenotype. Cancer Epidemiol Biomarkers Prev 2002;11:177–85.
[61] Naumburg E, Bellocco R, Cnattingius S, et al. Intrauterine exposure to diagnostic X-rays and risk of childhood leukemia subtypes. Radiat Res 2001;156:718–23.

[62] Shu XO, Reaman GH, Lampkin B, et al. Association of prenatal diagnostic x-ray exposure with risk of infant leukemia. Cancer Epidemiol Biomarkers Prev 1994;3:645–53.

[63] Whileman DC, Whileman CA, Green AC. Childhood sun exposure as risk factor for melanoma: a systematic review of epidemiological studies. Cancer Causes Control 2001;12(1): 69–82.

[64] Armstrong BC, Kricker A. The epidemiology of UV induced skin cancer. J Photochem Photobiol B 2001;63:8–18.

[65] Strouse JJ, Fears TR, Tucker M, et al. Pediatric melanoma: risk factor and survival analysis of the surveillance, epidemiological and end result database. J Clin Oncol 2005;23:4735–41.

[66] De Ross AJ, Teschke K, Savitz DA, et al. Parental occupational exposures to electric fields and radiation and the incidence of neuroblastoma in offspring. Epidemiology 2001;12: 508–17.

[67] Tardon A, Velarde H, Rodriquez P, et al. Exposure to extremely low frequency magnetic fields among primary school children in Spain. J Epidemiol Community Health 2002;56: 432–3.

[68] Dreadman JE, Armstrong BG, McBride ML, et al. Exposures of children in Canada to 60-HZ magnetic and electric fields. Scand J Work Environ Health 1999;25(4):368–75.

[69] Green LM, Millar AB, Agnew DA, et al. Childhood leukemia and personal monitoring of residential exposures to electric and magnetic fields in Ontario, Canada. Cancer Causes Control 1999;10(3):233–43.

[70] Green LM, Miller AB, Villeneuve PJ, et al. A case-control study of childhood leukemia in southern Ontario, Canada, and exposure to magnetic fields in residences. Int J Cancer 1999; 82:161–70.

[71] Draper G, Vincent T, Kroll ME, et al. Childhood cancer in relation to distance from high voltage power lines in England and Wales: a case-control study. BMJ 2005;330:1290. Avaliable at: http://www.bmj.com. Accessed at February 16, 2005.

[72] Linet MS, Hatch EE, Kleinerman RA, et al. Residential exposure to magnetic and acute lymphoblastic leukemia in children. N Engl J Med 1997;337:1–7.

[73] Kleinerman RA, Kaune WT, Hatch EE, et al. Are children living near high-voltage power lines at increased risk of acute lymphoblastic leukemia. Am J Epidemiol 2000;151:512–5.

[74] Li C, Lee W, Lin RS. Risk of leukemia in children living near high-voltage transmission lines. J Occup Environ Med 1998;40(2):144–7.

[75] Petridou E, Trichopoulos D, Kravaritis A, et al. Electrical power lines and childhood leukemia: a study from Greece. Int J Cancer 1997;73:345–8.

[76] Skinner J, Maslanyi MP, Mee TJ, et al. Childhood cancer and residential proximity to power lines. Br J Cancer 2000;83(11):1573–80.

[77] Feychting M, Floderus B, Ahlbom A. Parental occupational exposure to magnetic fields and childhood cancer (Sweden). Cancer Causes Control 2000;11:151–6.

[78] Infante-Rivard C, Deadman JE. Maternal occupation exposure to extremely low frequency magnetic fields during pregnancy and childhood leukemia. Epidemiology 2003;14:437–41.

[79] Preston-Martin S, Gurney JG, Pogoda JM, et al. Brain tumor risk in children in relation to use of electric blankets an water bed heaters. Am J Epidemiol 1996;143:1116–22.

[80] Soderberg KC, Naumburg E, Anger G, et al. Childhood leukemia and magnetic fields in infant incubators. Epidemiology 2002;13:45–9.

[81] Bianchl N, Crosignani P, Rovelli A, et al. Overhead electricity power lines and childhood leukemia: a registry-based, case-control study. Tumori 2000;86:195–8.

[82] Ni Y, Chang M, Wang K, et al. Clinical relevance of hepatitis B virus genotype in children with chronic infection and hepatocellular carcinoma. Gastroenterology 2004;127:1733–8.

[83] Lanier AP, Holek P, Day GE, et al. Childhood cancer among Alaska natives. Pediatrics 2003;112:396–403.

[84] Jarrett R. Risk factors for Hodgkin's lymphoma by EBV status and significance of detection of EBV genomes in serum of patients with EBV-associated Hodgkin's lymphoma. Leuk Lymphoma 2003;44(Suppl):S27–32.

[85] Chang MH, Shau WY, Chen CJ, et al. Hepatitis B vaccination and hepatocellular carcinoma rates in boys and girls. JAMA 2000;284:3040–2.

[86] Chen S, Chen C, Chou S, et al. Association of aflatoxin B_1-albumin adduct levels with hepatitis B surface antigen status among adolescents in Taiwan. Cancer Epidemiol Biomarkers Prev 2001;10:1223–6.

[87] Ming L, Thorgeirsson SS, Gail MH, et al. Dominant role of hepatitis B virus and cofactor role of aflatoxin in hepatocarcinogenesis in Qidong, China. Hepatology 2002;36(5):1046–9.

[88] Chang KC, Khen NT, Jones D, et al. Epstein-Barr virus associated with all histological subtypes of Hodgkin lymphoma in Vietnamese children with special emphasis on the entity of lymphocyte predominance subtypes. Hum Pathol 2005;36(7):747–55.

[89] De Matteo E, Baron AV, Chabay P, et al. Comparison of Epstein-Barr virus presence in Hodgkin lymphoma in pediatric versus adult Argentine patients. Arch Pathol Lab Med 2003;127(10):1325–9.

[90] Chabay P, De Matteo E, Merediz A, et al. High frequency of Epstein-Barr virus latent protein-1 30bp deletion in a series of pediatric malignancies in Argentina. Arch Virol 2004; 149(8):1515–26.

[91] Zhou XG, Sandveij K, Li PJ, et al. Epstein-Barr virus in Chinese pediatric Hodgkin disease: Hodgkin disease in young children is an EBV-related lymphoma. Cancer 2001;15(6): 1621–31.

[92] Kim SH, Shin YK, Lee IS, et al. Viral latent membrane protein 1(LMP-1)-induced CD down regulation in B cells leads to the generation of cells with Hodgkin's and Reed-Sternberg phenotype. Blood 2000;95(1):294–300.

[93] Drouet E, Brousset P, Fares F, et al. High Epstein-Barr virus serum load and elevated titters of anti-ZEBRA antibodies in patients with EBV-harboring tumor cells of Hodgkin's disease. J Med Virol 1999;57(4):383–9.

[94] Chang KL, Albujar PF, Chen YY, et al. High prevalence of Epstein-Barr virus in the Reed-Sternberg cells of Hodgkin's disease occurring in Peru. Blood 1993;81(2):496–501.

[95] Razzouk BL, Gan YJ, Mendonca C, et al. Epstein-Barr virus in pediatric Hodgkin disease: age and histiotype are more predictive than geographic region. Med Pediatr Oncol 1997; 28(4):248–54.

[96] Andriko JA, Aguilera NS, Nandedkar MA, et al. Childhood Hodgkin's in the United States: an analysis of histology subtypes and association with Epstein-Barr virus. Mod Pathol 1997;10(4):366–71.

[97] Weinreb M, Day PJ, Niggli F, et al. The consistent association between Epstein-Barr virus and Hodgkin's disease in children in Kenya. Blood 1996;87(9):3828–36.

[98] Moormann AM, Chelimo K, Sumba OP, et al. Exposure to holoendemic malaria results in elevated Epstein-Barr virus loads in children. J Infect Dis 2005;191(8):1233–8.

[99] Peh SC, Nadarajah VS, Tai YC, et al. Pattern of Epstein-Barr virus association in childhood non-Hodgkin's lymphoma: experience of university of Malaya medical center. Pathol Int 2004;54(3):151–7.

[100] Rasti N, Falk Ki, Donati D, et al. Circulatory Epstein-Barr virus in children living in malaria-endemic areas. Scand J Immunol 2005;61(5):461–5.

[101] Caterino-de-Araujo A, Cibella SE. Searching for antibodies to HHV-8 in children born to HIV-1 infected mothers from Sao Paulo, Brazil: relationship to maternal infection. J Trop Pediatr 2003;49(4):247–50.

[102] Chakraborty R, Rees G, Bourboulia D, et al. Viral coinfection among African children infected with human immunodeficiency virus type 1. Clin Infect Dis 2003;36(7):922–4.

[103] Caseli D, Klersy C, de Martino MD, et al. Human immunodeficiency virus-related cancer in the Italian register. J Clin Oncol 2000;18:3854–61.

[104] Evans JA, Gibb DM, Holland FJ, et al. Malignancies in UK children with HIV infection acquired from mother to child transmission. Arch Dis Child 1997;76:330–3.

[105] Biggar RJ, Frisch M, Goedert JJ, et al. Risk of cancer in children with AIDS. JAMA 2000; 284:205–9.

[106] Mueller BU, Pizza PA. Malignancies in pediatric AIDS. Curr Opin Pediatr 1996;8:45–9.
[107] Bourugian MJ, Spinelli JJ, Mezei G, et al. Childhood leukemia and socioeconomic status in Canada. Epidemiology 2005;16(4):526–31.
[108] Karimi M, Yarmohammadi H. Seasonal variations in the onset of childhood leukemia/lymphoma: April 1996 to March 2000, Shiraz, Iran. Hematol Oncol 2003;21:51–5.
[109] Felltbower RG, Peace MS, Dickenson HO, et al. Seasonality of birth for cancer in Northern England, UK. Paediatr Perinat Epidemiol 2001;15:338–45.
[110] Kinlen LJ, Balkwill A. Infective cause of childhood leukemia and wartime population mixing in Orkney and Shetland, UK. Lancet 2001;357(9529):858.
[111] McNally RJQ, Eden TOB, Alexander FE, et al. Is there a common aetiology for certain childhood malignancies? Results of cross-space-time clustering analyses. Eur J Cancer 2005;41(18):2911–6.
[112] Health CW Jr. Community clusters of childhood leukemia and lymphoma: evidence of infection? Am J Epidemiol 2005;162:1–6.
[113] Greaves M. Speculation on the cause of childhood acute lymphoblastic leukemia. Leukemia 1988;2:120–5.
[114] Kinlen L. Evidence for an infective cause of childhood leukemia: comparison of a Scottish New Town with nuclear reprocessing sites in Britain. Lancet 1988;2(8624):1323–7.
[115] Kinlen L. Epidemiological evidence for an infective basis in childhood leukemia. Br J Cancer 1995;71:1–5.
[116] Smith M. Considerations on a possible viral etiology for B-precursor acute lymphoblastic leukemia of childhood. J Immunol 1997;20:89–100.
[117] Taub JW, Konrad MA, Ge Y, et al. High frequency of leukemic clones in newborn screening blood samples of children with B-precursor acute lymphoblastic leukemia. Blood 2002;99(8):2992–6.
[118] Dockerty JD, Skeg DCG, Elwood JM, et al. Infections, vaccinations, and the risk of childhood leukemia. Br J Cancer 1999;80(9):1483–9.
[119] Perrillat F, Clavel J, Auclerc MF, et al. Day-care, early common infections and childhood acute leukemia: a multicentre French case—control study. Br J Cancer 2002;86:1064–9.
[120] Gilham C, Peto J, Simpson J, et al. Day care in infancy and risk of childhood acute lymphoblastic leukemia: findings from UK case-control study. BMJ 2005;330:1294–300.
[121] Kwan ML, Buffler PA, Abrams B, et al. Breastfeeding and the risk of childhood leukemia: a meta-analysis. Public Health Rep 2004;119:521–35.
[122] Jourdan-Da Silva N, Perel Y, Mechinaud F, et al. Infectious diseases in the first year of life, perinatal characteristics and childhood acute leukemia. Br J Cancer 2004;90:139–45.
[123] Infante-Rivard C, Firtier I, Olson F. Markers of infection, breast-feeding and childhood acute lymphoblastic leukemia. Br J Cancer 2000;83:1559–64.
[124] Alexander FE, Chan LC, Lam TH, et al. Clustering of childhood leukemia in Hong Kong: association with the childhood peak and common acute lymphoblastic leukemia and with population mixing. Br J Cancer 1997;75(3):457–63.
[125] Raaschou-Nielsen O, Obel J, Dalton S, et al. Socioeconomic status and risk of childhood leukemia in Denmark. Scand J Public Health 2004;32:279–86.
[126] Pearce MS, Cotterill SJ, Parker L. Father's occupational contacts and risk of childhood leukemia and non-Hodgkin lymphoma. Epidemiology 2004;15:352–6.
[127] Kinlen LJ, Bramald S. Paternal occupational contact level and childhood leukemia in rural Scotland. Br J Cancer 2001;84:1002–7.
[128] McNally RJQ, Eden TOB. An infectious etiology for childhood acute leukaemia: a review of the evidence. Br J Haematol 2004;127:243–63.
[129] International Agency for Research on Cancer (IARC). Diesel and gasoline exhaust and some nitroarenes. IARC Monogr Eval Carcinog Risks Hum 1989;46:41–185.
[130] Perera F, Hemminki K, Jedrychowski W, et al. In utero DNA damage from environmental pollution is associated with somatic gene mutation in newborns. Cancer Epidemiol Biomarkers Prev 2002;11:1134–7.

[131] Pahjala SK, Lappi M, Hankanen M, et al. Comparison of mutagenicity and calf thymus DNA adducts formed by the particulate and semivolatile fractions of vehicle exhausts. Environ Mol Mutagen 2003;42:26–36.

[132] Lin Y, Keane M, Ensell M, et al. In vitro genotoxicity of exhaust emissions of diesel and gasoline engine vehicle on a united driving cycle. J Environ Monit 2005;7: 60–6.

[133] Bocskay KA, Tang D, Orjucla MA, et al. Chromosomal aberrations in cord blood are associated with prenatal exposure to carcinogenic polycyclic aromatic hydrocarbons. Cancer Epidemiol Biomarkers Prev 2005;14(2):506–11.

[134] Reynolds P, Behren JV, Gunier RB, et al. Traffic patterns and childhood cancer incidence in California, United States. Cancer Causes Control 2002;13:665–73.

[135] Savitz DA, Feingold L. Association of childhood cancer with traffic density. Scand J Work Environ Health 1989;15:360–3.

[136] Reynolds P, Elkin Eric, Scalf R, et al. A case-control pilot study of traffic exposures and early childhood leukemia using a geographic information system. Bioelectromagnetics 2001;22(Suppl 5):S58–68.

[137] Pearson RL, Wachtchel H, Ebi KL. Distance-weighted traffic density in proximity to a home is a risk for leukemia and other childhood cancers. J Air Waste Manage Assoc 2000;50:175–80.

[138] Harrison RM, Leung PL, Somervaille L, et al. Analysis of childhood cancer in the West Midlands of the United Kingdom in relation to proximity to main roads and petrol stations. Occup Environ Med 1999;56:774–80.

[139] Steffen C, Auclerc MF, Auvrognon A, et al. Acute childhood leukemia and environmental exposure to potential sources of benzene and other hydrocarbons; a case-control study. Occup Environ Med 2004;61:773–8.

[140] Crosignani P, Tittarelli A, Borgini A, et al. Childhood leukemia and road traffic: a population-based case-control study. Int J Cancer 2004;108:596–9.

[141] Feychting M, Svensson D, Ahlbom A. Exposure to motor vehicle exhaust and childhood cancer. Scand J Work Environ Health 1998;24(1):8–11.

[142] Raaschou-Nielsen O, Hertel O, Thomsen BL, et al. Air pollution from traffic at the residence of children with cancer. Am J Epidemiol 2001;153:433–43.

[143] Knox EG. Oil combustion and childhood cancers. J Epidemiol Community Health 2005; 59(9):755–60.

[144] Knox EG. Childhood cancers and atmospheric carcinogens. J Epidemiol Community Health 2005;59:101–5.

[145] Reynolds P, Behren JV, Gunier RB, et al. Childhood cancer incidence rates and hazardous air pollutants in California; an exploratory analysis. Environ Health Perspect 2003;111: 663–8.

[146] Sasco AJ, Secretan MB, Straif K. Tobacco smoking and cancer: a brief review of recent epidemiological evidence. Lung Cancer 2004;45(Suppl):S3–9.

[147] Brennan P, Buffer PA, Reynolds P, et al. Second hand smoke exposure in adulthood and risk of lung cancer among never smokers: a pooled analysis of two large studies. Int J Cancer 2004;109(1):125–31.

[148] Filippini G, Maisonneuve P, McCredie M, et al. Relation of childhood brain tumors to exposure of parents and children to tobacco smoke: the SEARCH international case-control study. Surveillance of environmental aspects related to cancer in humans. Int J Cancer 2002;100(2):206–13.

[149] Hu J, Mao Y, Ugnat AM. Parental cigarette smoking, hard liquor consumption and the risk of childhood brain tumors—a case control study in northeast China. Acta Oncol 2000;39(8):979–84.

[150] Brooks DR, Mucci LA, Hatch EE, et al. Maternal smoking during pregnancy and risk of brain tumors in the offspring. A prospective study of 1.4 million Swedish births. Cancer Causes Control 2004;15:997–1005.

[151] Boffeta P, Trendaniel J, Grecco A. Risk of childhood cancer and adult lung cancer after childhood exposure to passive smoke: a meta-analysis. Environ Health Perspect 2000; 108(1):73–82.

[152] Infante-Rivard C, Krajinivic M, Labuda D, et al. Parental smoking, CYP1A1 genetic polymorphism and childhood leukemia (Quebec, Canada). Cancer Causes Control 2000;11(6): 547–53.

[153] Brondum J, Shu XO, Steinbuch M, et al. Parental cigarette smoking and risk of acute leukemia in children. Cancer 1999;85(6):1380–8.

[154] Sorahan T, Prior P, Lancashire RJ, et al. Childhood cancer and parental use of tobacco: deaths from 1971 to 1976. Br J Cancer 1997;76(11):1523–31.

[155] Filippini G, Farinotti M, Ferrarini M. Active and passive smoking during pregnancy and risk of central nervous system tumors in children. Paediatr Perinat Epidemiol 2000;14(1):78–84.

[156] Severson RK, Buckley JD, Woods WG, et al. Cigarette smoking and alcohol consumption by parents of children with acute myeloid leukemia: an analysis within morphological subgroups- a report from the Children's Cancer Group. Cancer Epidemiol Biomarkers Prev 1993;2(5):433–9.

[157] Chen Z, Robinson L, Giller R, et al. Risk of childhood germ cell tumors in association with parental smoking and drinking. Cancer 2005;103(5):1064–71.

[158] Shu XO, Nesbit ME, Buckley JD, et al. An exploratory analysis of risk factors for childhood malignant germ-cell tumors: report from the Children's Cancer Group (Canada, United States). Cancer Causes Control 1995;6(3):187–98.

[159] Sorahan T, Lancashire RJ. Parental cigarette smoking and childhood risks of hepatoblastoma: OSCC data. Br J Cancer 2004;90(5):10016–8.

[160] Buckley JD, Sather H, Ruccione K, et al. A case-control study of risk factors for hepatoblastoma. A report from the Children's Cancer Study Group. Cancer 1989;64(5):1169–76.

[161] Husgafvel-Pursiainen K. Genotoxicity of environmental tobacco smoke: a review. Mutat Res 2004;567(2–3):527–45.

[162] Grant SG. Qualitatively and quantitatively similar effects of active and passive maternal tobacco exposure on in utero mutagenesis at the HPRT locus. BMC Pediatrics 2005;5:20. Available at: http://www.biomedcentral.com/1471-231/5/20. Accessed February 17, 2006.

[163] Bishun NP, Smith NS, Williams DC, et al. Carcinogenic and possible mutagenic effects of Stilboestrol in offspring exposed in utero. J Surg Oncol 1977;9:293–300.

[164] Wen W, Shu XO, Potter JD, et al. Parental medication use and risk of childhood acute lymphoblastic leukemia. Cancer 2002;95(8):1786–94.

[165] Kwan ML, Block G, Selvin S, et al. Food consumption by children and the risk of childhood acute leukemia. Am J Epidemiol 2004;160:1098–107.

[166] Peters JM, Preston-Martin S, London SJ, et al. Processed meats and risk of childhood leukemia (California, USA). Cancer Causes Control 1994;5:195–202.

[167] Infante-Rivard C, Olson E, Jacques L, et al. Drinking water contaminants and childhood leukemia. Epidemiology 2001;12(1):13–9.

[168] Huncharek M, Kupelnick B. A meta-analysis of maternal cured meat consumption during pregnancy and the risk of childhood brain tumors. Neuroepidemiology 2004;23: 78–84.

[169] Robison LL, Buckley JD, Daigle AE, et al. Maternal drug use and risk of childhood nonlymphoblastic leukemia among offspring. An epidemiologic investigation implicating marijuana (A Report from the Children's Cancer Study Group). Cancer 1989;63: 1904–11.

[170] Grufferman S, Grossbart Schwartz A, Ruymann FB, et al. Parents' use of cocaine and marijuana and increased risk of rhabdomyosarcoma in their children. Cancer Causes Control 1993;4:217–24.

[171] Flower KB, Hoppin JA, Lynch CF, et al. Cancer risk and parental pesticide application in children of agricultural health study participants. Environ Health Perspect 2004;112(5): 631–5.

[172] Ma X, Buffler PA, Gunier RB, et al. Critical windows of exposure to household pesticides and risk of childhood leukemia. Environ Health Perspect 2002;110(9):955–60.

[173] Valery PC, McWhirter W, Sleigh A, et al. Farm exposures, parental occupation, and risk of Ewing's sarcoma in Australia: a national case-control study. Cancer Causes Control 2002; 13:263–70.

[174] vanWijngaarden E, Stewart PA, Olshan AF, et al. Parental occupational exposure to pesticides and childhood brain cancer. Am J Epidemiol 2003;157:989–97.

[175] Daniels JL, Olshan AF, Savitz DA. Pesticides and childhood cancers. Environ Health Perspect 1997;105(10):1068–77.

[176] Schuz J, Kaletsch U, Meinert R, et al. Risk of childhood leukemia and parental self-reported occupational exposure to chemicals, dusts, and fumes: results from pooled analyses of German population-based case-control studies. Cancer Epidemiol Biomarkers Prev 2000;9:835–8.

[177] Infante-Rivard C, Siemiatycki J, Lakhani R, et al. Maternal exposure to occupational solvents and childhood leukemia. Environ Health Perspect 2005;113(6):787–92.

[178] Cordier S, Mandereau L, Preston-Martin S, et al. Parental occupations and childhood brain tumors: results of an international case-control study. Cancer Causes Control 2001; 12:865–74.

[179] De Roos AJ, Olshan AF, Teschke K, et al. Parental occupational exposures to chemicals and incidence of neuroblastoma in offspring. Am J Epidemiol 2001;154(2):106–14.

[180] Heeg S, Doebele M, von Werder A, Opitz OG. In vitro transformation models: modeling human cancer. Cell Cycle 2006;5(6):630–4.

[181] Kraemer KH, Lee MM, Andrews AD, et al. The role of sunlight and DNA repair in melanoma and nonmelanoma skin cancer. The xeroderma pigmentosum paradigm. Arch Dermatol 1994;130:1018–21.

[182] Plon SE, Nathanson K. Inherited susceptibility for pediatric cancer. Cancer J 2005;11(4): 255–67.

[183] Ross JA, Potter JD, Reaman GH, et al. Maternal exposure to potential inhibitors of DNA topoisomerase II and infant leukemia (United States): a report from the children's cancer group. Cancer Causes Control 1996;7:581–90.

[184] Ross JA. Maternal diet and infant leukemia: a role for DNA topoisomerase II inhibitors? Int J Cancer(Suppl) 1998;11:26–8.

[185] Krajinovic M, Richer C, Sinnett H, et al. Genetic polymorphisms of N-acetyltransferases 1 and 2 and gene-gene interaction in the susceptibility to childhood acute lymphoblastic leukemia. Cancer Epidemiol Biomarkers Prev 2000;9:557–62.

[186] Krajinovic M, Sinnett H, Richer C, et al. Role of NQOI, MPO and CYP2E1 genetic polymorphisms in the susceptibility to childhood acute lymphoblastic leukemia. Int J Cancer 2002;97:230–6.

[187] Canalle R, Burim RV, Tone LG, et al. Genetic polymorphisms and susceptibility to childhood acute lymphoblastic leukemia. Environ Mol Mutagen 2004;43:100–9.

[188] Searles Nielsen S, Mueller BA, De Roos AJ, et al. Risk of brain tumors in children and susceptibility to organophosphorus insecticides: the potential role of paraoxonase (PON1). Environ Health Perspect 2005;113:909–13.

[189] Tokunaga M, Norman JE Jr, Asano M, et al. Malignant breast tumors among atomic bomb survivors, Hiroshima and Nagasaki, 1954–1974. J Natl Cancer Inst 1979;62(6): 1347–59.

[190] Tokunaga M, Land CE, Yamamoto T, et al. Incidence of female breast cancer among atomic bomb survivors, Hiroshima and Nagasaki, 1950–1980. Radiat Res 1987;112(2): 243–72.

[191] Land CE, Tokunaga M, Koyama K, et al. Incidence of female breast cancer among atomic bomb survivors, Hiroshima and Nagasaki, 1950–1990. Radiat Res 2003;160(6):707–17.

[192] Ron E, Preston DL, Kishikawa M, et al. Skin tumor risk among atomic-bomb survivors in Japan. Cancer Causes Control 1998;9(4):393–401.

[193] Preston DL, Ron E, Yonehara S, et al. Tumors of the nervous system and pituitary gland associated with atomic bomb radiation exposure. J Natl Cancer Inst 2002;94(20):1555–63.

[194] Thompson DE, Mabuchi K, Ron E, et al. Cancer incidence in atomic bomb survivors. Part II: solids tumors, 1958–1987. Radiat Res 1994;137(2 Suppl):S17–67.

[195] Guiboul C, Adjadi E, Rubino C, et al. Malignant breast tumors after radiotherapy for a first cancer during childhood. J Clin Oncol 2005;23:197–204.

[196] Sadetzki S, Chetrit A, Freedman L, et al. Long-tern follow-up for brain tumor development after childhood exposure to ionizing radiation for tinea capitis. Radiat Res 2005;163: 424–32.

[197] Vega-Stromberg T. Chemotherapy-induced secondary malignancies. J Infus Nurs 2003; 26(6):353–60.

[198] Naldi L, Altieri A, Imberti GL, et al. Sun exposure, phenotypic characteristics, and cutaneous malignant melanoma. An analysis according to different clinico-pathological variants and anatomic locations (Italy). Cancer Causes Control 2005;16(8):893–9.

[199] Gallagher RP, Spinelli JJ, Lee TK. Tanning beds, sunlamps, and risks of cutaneous malignant melanoma. Cancer Epidemiol Biomarkers Prev 2005;14(3):562–6.

[200] Siskind V, Aitken J, Green A, et al. Sun exposure and interaction with family history of melanoma, Queensland, Australia. Int J Cancer 2002;97(1):90–5.

[201] Autier P, Dore JF. Influence of sun exposures during childhood and during adulthood on melanoma risk. EPIMEL and EORTC Melanoma Cooperative Group. European Organization for Research and Treatment of Cancer. Int J Cancer 1998;77(4):533–7.

[202] Vineis P, Airoldi L, Vegilla F, et al. Environmental tobacco smoke and risk of respiratory cancer and chronic obstructive pulmonary disease in former smokers and never smokers in the EPIC prospective study. BMJ 2005;330:277.

[203] Okasha M, McCarron P, Gunnel D, et al. Exposures in childhood, adolescence and early adulthood and breast cancer risk; a systematic review of the literature. Breast Cancer Res Treat 2003;78(2):223–76.

[204] Bonner MR, Nie D, Han D, et al. Secondhand smoke exposure in early life and the risk of breast cancer among never smokers (United States). Cancer Causes Control 2005;16(6): 683–9.

[205] Sandler DP, Wilcox AJ, Eyerson RB. Cumulative effects of lifetime passive smoking on cancer risk. Lancet 1985;1(8424):1312–5.

[206] Sandler DP, Eyerson RB, Wilcox AJ, et al. Cancer risk in adult from early life exposure to parents smoking. Am J Public Health 1985;73:487–92.

[207] Yang XR, Diehl S, Pfeiffer R, et al. Evaluation of risk factors for nasopharyngeal carcinoma in high-risk nasopharyngeal carcinoma in Taiwan. Cancer Epidemiol Biomarkers Prev 2005;14(4):900–5.

[208] Abdulrazzag YM, Osman N, Yousif ZM, et al. Aflatoxin M_1 in breastmilk of UAE women. Annals of Tropical Paediatrics: International Child Health 2003;23:173–9.

[209] Wild CP, Yin F, Turner PC, et al. Environmental and genetic determinant of aflatoxin-albumin adducts in the Gambia. Int J Cancer 2000;86(1):1–7.

[210] Wei WI, Sham JS. Nasopharyngeal carcinoma. Lancet 2005;365(9476):2041–54.

ELSEVIER
SAUNDERS

Pediatr Clin N Am
54 (2007) 205–212

PEDIATRIC CLINICS
OF NORTH AMERICA

Index

Note: Page numbers of article titles are in **boldface** type.

A

Acid mine water, environmental pollution by, 155–156

Adhesive exposures, epidemiology of, 18, 22

Agency for Toxic Substances and Disease Registry, 2. *See also* Pediatric Environmental Health Specialty Units Program.
exposure data from, 15, 28
website of, 135, 137, 145

Agricultural environment, health issues in, 123–124, 126–127

Air pollution
asthma due to, 108–114
cancer due to, 183–185, 190
in rural environment, 122–123, 128
risk communication about, 33–46

Alcohol ingestion
developmental disabilities due to, 51–52
epidemiology of, 21–22, 24–25

Aldrin, Stockholm Convention and, 85

Alkali exposures, epidemiology of, 24

All terrain vehicles, injuries from, 124–125

Allergens, in asthma
cat, 106–107, 109
cockroach, 105–106, 109
dog, 106–107, 109
dust mite, 104–105, 109
rodent, 107–109

American Academy of Pediatrics, environmental health information from, 139, 149

American Association of Poison Control Centers, data from, in epidemiologic studies, 16–17, 19–21, 24–25, 28–29

America's Children & the Environment, 147

Animals, injuries from, in rural environment, 124, 128

Arsenic exposure
absorption in, selenium and, 165
epidemiology of, 18
neurotoxicity in, 160–161, 163

Arts and crafts supply exposures, epidemiology of, 19–20, 22

Association of Occupational and Environmental Clinics, 2–3, 11, 17

Asthma, environmental influences on, **103–120**
carbon monoxide, 113
cat allergens, 106–107, 109
cockroach allergens, 105–106, 109
dog allergens, 106–107, 109
dust mite allergens, 104–105, 109
nitrogen dioxide, 111–112
ozone, 110
particulate matter, 110–111
pesticides, 76
rodent allergens, 107–109
sulfur dioxide, 113
tobacco smoke, 112–113

Atomic bomb radiation exposure, cancer after, 177–178

Attention deficit hyperactivity disorder
environmental etiologies of, 50–52
counseling on, 59–60
evaluation in, 52–57
treatment of, 57–59
epidemiology of, 49–50

Autistic spectrum disorder
environmental etiologies of, 50–52
counseling on, 59–60
evaluation in, 52–57
treatment of, 57–59
epidemiology of, 49

B

Battery exposure, epidemiology of, 23–24

Birth defects, from pesticide exposure, 74–75

Bleach exposure, epidemiology of, 19–20, 24

doi:10.1016/S0031-3955(07)00021-1
pediatric.theclinics.com

developmental disabilities due to,
51–52
endocrine disruption in, 87–88
epidemiology of, 18, 22, 24
family questions on, 76–78
high-risk populations for, 73–74
in food, 73
information resources for,
70–71, 148
occupational, 73
Stockholm Convention and, 84–85
symptoms of, 65–69

Phosphonate exposures, symptoms of, 68

Picher Lead/Zinc Mining District (Tar
Creek Superfund site), mining wastes
in, 157–161, 165

Plant exposures, epidemiology of, 19–20,
22, 24–25

Polish exposure, epidemiology of,
18, 22

Polybrominated diphenyl ether exposure,
90–91, 95

Polychlorinated biphenyl exposure
developmental disabilities due to, 51
health effects of, 86–89
Stockholm Convention and, 85–86

Polycyclic aromatic hydrocarbon exposures,
cancer in, 185–187, 192

Pregnancy, environmental exposures in
cancer in, 179–180, 182, 184–185,
187–193
developmental disabilities due to,
50–52, 55
infectious agents, 184–185
mining wastes, 161–163
occupational, 189
persistent organic pollutants, 86–89
pesticides, 75, 188–189
radiation, 179–180, 182
substances of abuse, 188
tobacco smoke, 187

Pyrethrin exposure, 66–67, 69

R

Radiation exposure, cancer in
adult-onset, 191
high-dose ionizing, 179–180
low-dose ionizing, 180–182
non-ionizing, 182–183

Radiography, cancer due to, 182

Radon exposure, cancer in, 181, 192

Rat allergens, in asthma, 107–109

Risk communication, in environmental
health, **33–46**
case study of, 39–44
cognitive attenuation in, 37
importance of, 33–34
message development for, 37–39
practical application of, 44–46
principles of, 34–37
risk perception in, 34–36
Seven Cardinal Rules of, 44–45
trust determination in, 36

Rodent allergens, in asthma, 107–109

Rodenticide exposures
epidemiology of, 19–20
symptoms of, 68

Rule of three, for risk communication
message, 37

Rural environment, health issues in,
121–133
agriculture-related problems,
126–127
air quality, 122–123, 128
animal-related injuries, 124, 128
demographics of, 122
drowning, 125, 129
epidemiology of, 26–27
firearm injuries, 124
information resources for, 128–129
mortality, 122
motor vehicle injuries, 124–125, 128
obesity, 125–126, 129
occupational injuries, 127, 129
pesticides, 126–127
water quality, 123, 128

S

Scabicide exposures, 69

Scorecard website, 151

Selenium, arsenic absorption and, 167

Skin cancer, from radiation exposure, 182

Smoke exposure
asthma in, 112–113
cancer in, 187, 191–193
epidemiology of, 23

Soap exposures, epidemiology of, 19–20

Soil toxin exposures, epidemiology of, 18

Solar radiation exposure, cancer in, 182,
191, 193

Stockholm Convention on Persistent
Organic Pollutants, 82, 84–86

Sulfur dioxide exposure, asthma in, 113

Moving?

Make sure your subscription moves with you!

To notify us of your new address, find your **Clinics Account Number** (located on your mailing label above your name), and contact customer service at:

E-mail: elspcs@elsevier.com

800-654-2452 (subscribers in the U.S. & Canada)
407-345-4000 (subscribers outside of the U.S. & Canada)

Fax number: 407-363-9661

Elsevier Periodicals Customer Service
6277 Sea Harbor Drive
Orlando, FL 32887-4800

*To ensure uninterrupted delivery of your subscription, please notify us at least 4 weeks in advance of move.